Pelican Books
Drugs

Peter Laurie was born in Reigate in 1937. His father was an inventor, and his mother the daughter of an American journalist. He had what he describes as a conventional middle-class education at Lancing and Cambridge University, where he read mathematics and law. At Cambridge he started the picture magazine *Image*, and consequently he was hired by *Vogue* on the wave of the Cambridge satirists. During his three years at *Vogue* he contributed also to the *Daily Mail* and the *Sunday Telegraph*. Then after three weeks as assistant editor of the *Weekend Telegraph* he became editor of *Town*. He is now a freelance journalist working mainly for the *Sunday Times Magazine*. He says he finds magazine journalism the perfect life because it offers the opportunity to become deeply but temporarily involved in the lives of interesting people, and he feels that there is at least an important role for the intellectual dilettante who tries to inform the world of what is happening in the increasingly complex fields of science and social policy. His book *Teenage Revolution* was published in 1965, and *Scotland Yard* in 1969. *Beneath the City Streets*, a study of Civil Defence, was published by Allen Lane in 1970.

Peter Laurie was married at twenty-one, and he now lives in Paddington with his wife and three children.

Peter Laurie

Drugs

Medical, Psychological and Social Facts

Penguin Books

Penguin Books Ltd, Harmondsworth,
Middlesex, England
Penguin Books, 625 Madison Avenue,
New York, New York 10022, U.S.A.
Penguin Books Australia Ltd, Ringwood,
Victoria, Australia
Penguin Books Canada Ltd, 2801 John Street,
Markham, Ontario, Canada L3R 1B4
Penguin Books (N.Z.) Ltd, 182–190 Wairau Road,
Auckland 10, New Zealand

First published 1967
Reprinted 1967 (three times), 1968
Reissued as a Pelican 1969
Reprinted 1969, 1970
Second edition 1971
Reprinted 1972
Reprinted with revisions 1974
Reprinted 1976
Reprinted with revisions 1978
Reprinted 1979

Made and printed in Great Britain by
C. Nicholls & Company Ltd
Set in Monotype Times

Contents

Preface

This book is a crude attempt to sum up the major points of our knowledge, and still more our ignorance, about drugs; how to define and control the harm they do to personalities and to society. It is not intended as a handbook on even the small number of drugs that are mentioned, but rather as the beginnings of a rational discussion of drugs in society, and the vehicle for putting forward some new attitudes towards them. If it appears superficial, it must be remembered that although perhaps 10,000 scientific papers have been published on this subject – 1,000 on the hallucinogens alone – in the last fifty years, there is an amazingly small amount of hard information available. Among scientists, as among laymen, this subject stimulates endless streams of subjective, narrative evidence, wild claims and repetitive accounts. My purpose has been to select and assemble some useful nuggets from this vast and amorphous mass. If the reader finishes this book feeling no wiser but rather more confused than before, he is in the same case as the honest professional. Of all the social problems drug abuse is the most intractable and inexplicable. No one in the world has an adequate answer.

It may be relevant to say something about my own attitude towards drugs. Apart from a couple of experiments with benzedrine at school in the mid fifties – during the inhaler craze – and two rather abortive experiences with L S D and marihuana reported here, I have not used drugs and I am not very tempted to. The society of drug users does not seem to me to be particularly interesting – probably my own fault – and life is too busy to afford the time necessary to get to know them. In general, I think, I am one of those people who is impaired by any drug. I do not smoke, and I seldom drink, at least seldom in comparison with my parents' generation.

Broadly speaking, commentators on drugs – both lay and

expert – tend to divide sharply into those who are basically pessimistic about humanity and think that drugs distort and corrupt personality, and the optimists who think that nothing, including drugs, changes people very much from their true reality. Both points of view are probably equally wrong, but I must admit to being among the second class.

It may seem impertinent for a journalist without any medical training to write on such a technical subject. My defences are that (a) this field covers so many disciplines that no single person is going to be professionally qualified to speak on them all, (b) in these days of experts, it is perhaps useful that uninformed, but also unindoctrinated persons should do a sort of consumer test on scientific work, reviewing what has been done, and asking: how far forward does this get society?

I have to thank many people: the librarians of the Wellcome, British Medical Association and Royal Society of Medicine libraries for allowing me to consult their shelves. I have to thank those addicts and doctors who talked to me, Commander Millen of the Metropolitan Police and other police officers with whom I had interviews when I wrote the first edition of this book in 1965. Finally I have to thank the staff of the Home Office Drugs Branch and Professor G. M. Carstairs of Edinburgh University, who all suggested several most useful lines of thought and inquiry and removed many of the crasser mistakes from my first manuscript. It would be beyond human power to remove them all.

Preface to the 1974 Edition

This edition appears at a time when the scientific arguments about drugs have almost died down. The major facts are no longer in dispute: the interesting research now being done is aimed at showing that drug use is compatible with productive conventional life (heroin, see p. 154; marihuana, p. 42). The battle has moved from the laboratory to the hustings: the forces opposed are becoming more and more political, and the issues at stake in the legalization of soft drugs are economic and social rather than moral or medical.

Two more important inquiries – the President's Committee on Marihuana and Drug Abuse in America, and the le Dain Commission in Canada – have reported that marihuana is not a significant social danger. Yet in both countries, as in Britain and many others too, legislation has become more severe and in America particularly vast sums are being spent to extirpate the drug traffic. President Nixon announced in 1973 a budget of $430 million to deal with the drug problem. When one realizes that this represents the salaries of 30,000 middle class administrators, the size of vested interests that are being installed against liberalization of the drug laws becomes apparent. One fears that the legislators are whistling in the dark, for illegal drug use has now become a habit indulged in by substantial numbers of people. A survey by the New York Chamber of Commerce found that of 579,000 sales people in the city, 12,000 were addicted to heroin, 21,000 to amphetamines, 50,000 to marihuana, 37,000 to tranquillizers, and 71,000 to barbiturates. A survey by the B.B.C. programme *Midweek* in 1973 found that 4 million people in Britain had smoked cannabis, 657,000 had tried LSD, 1.2 millions amphetamine, and that half a million people were addicted to barbiturates.

Again, I must thank all those who helped me to write this book and keep it moderately up to date, and in particular the staff of the Institute for the Study of Drug Dependence, whose excellent library made the task of revision very much easier.

1
The Meaning of Drug

For the purposes of this book, a *drug* is any chemical substance that alters mood, perception or consciousness and is misused, to the apparent detriment of society. We exclude alcohol as a drug because our society is itself dependent on it, and as Prohibition seems to have shown, its enforced absence is more damaging than its legal presence.

In many people's minds, the most important and dangerous quality of a drug is its *addictiveness*. To begin with semantics: there has been, and still is, a woolly debate about the proper words to apply to drug abuse. 'Addict' and its compounds are now out of fashion; but since the word still popularly encapsulates the menace, we will have to use it, but with reservations. In this work 'addict', 'addictive', 'addiction' and so on will only be applied to drugs that cause physical changes in the body, perpetuating their use. That is, 'tolerance' is established in the 'addict', and he needs more of the drug to hold off withdrawal symptoms or to reach the same intensity of effect.

It might be thought that here we have the problem nailed. Addictive drugs physically enslave; non-addictive drugs do not. Find an antidote or a harmless substitute and your drug problem is solved. Unfortunately it is all more complicated. The common addictive drugs are: alcohol, morphine, heroin and barbiturates. There are many examples of people who use them without becoming either physically or psychically dependent on them. There are also examples of people who become extremely dependent on drugs that cause no long-term changes in the body at all, like cannabis. But the distinction between physically addictive and non-addictive drugs is still worth making, if only for a negative reason: it doesn't very much matter.

The World Health Organization recommend saying 'drug dependence':

Individuals may become dependent on a wide variety of chemical substances covering the whole range of pharmacodynamic effects from stimulation to depression. All these drugs have this in common: they are capable of creating a state of mind in some individuals which is termed psychic dependence. This is a psychic drive which requires periodic or chronic administration of the substance for pleasure or to avoid discomfort. Indeed it is the most powerful factor involved in chronic intoxication with psychotropic drugs. With certain types of drugs it may be the only factor involved, even in the most intense types of craving and compulsive abuse.[1]

One might add that people become dependent not only on drugs but on the experiences drugs give, and indeed on experiences which are obtained quite independently of drugs. There are many in our society who need the satisfaction of fast driving as badly as many addicts need their drugs, and their 'fix' causes a good deal more social damage. We can see, when we think about him, that the delinquent driver is the product of opportunity, inadequate personality and bad training; but we like to look on the drug addict as the tragic victim of an irresistible delight.

The debate over 'addiction', 'habituation' and the fruitless inquiry whether this or that drug falls into one class or another was perhaps misconceived. It was supposed that a pharmacological peculiarity of some drugs made them either grip or not grip the system of their user. But how to explain the fact that many people can use heroin and give it up? (See p. 154.)

The experiments of Pavlov showed that any experience can be involuntarily and unconsciously associated in the mind with any other, providing one happens soon after the other. If conditions are right, the link can be extremely strong and durable, and each time it is repeated the bonds are strengthened. Thus when we come across someone who is said to be 'addicted' to a drug like marihuana which produces no physical habituation at all, in the sense that they demand it, say they can't live without it, are depressed when deprived of it, and so on (see p. 95 for an example) we have a situation which is a function of the pleasurable effects of the drug, the bleak inner life of the addict, the sympathetic social conditions under which he has used the drug. He has become conditioned in a Pavlovian way to the drug as a sole source of pleasure, and every time he proves himself right, his dependence is strengthened. At the same time, by being the sort of person he is, by leading the life he does, he makes the chances of learning new sources of gratification – from working well, having a stable relationship with a wife – more and more remote. This idea was proposed to explain the otherwise mysterious relapses of heroin addicts who, often decades after their cure, start using the drug again, when one would expect them to have every reason not to. The theory is that during their addiction they became conditioned to heroin as a reliever of anxiety. Whenever anything threatened them then they would give themselves a shot; years later when anxiety is strong enough it breaks through the later training against use.[2]

All that is necessary for conditioning and dependence is some effect from the drug. Since, by definition, any drug produces a mental effect, any drug can form dependence if experienced in the right way by the right person. But one need not confine the argument to chemicals taken internally. Clothes are artificial metabolic aids that satisfy many of the criteria for dependence-producing drugs. We all – all men that is – rely heavily on our trousers; if they are taken away, we can suffer disabling physical and mental stress. Shoes are another example. We even have a name for people who become unusually dependent on them: fetishists.

As a chart to the chapters ahead, a table follows, setting out the principal effects of the problem drugs, with a couple of other substances for the purposes of comparison.

The whole problem of drug effects and dependence is complicated by the effect of the social surroundings in which they are taken, and the expectations of those that use them. It is almost meaningless, particularly when one is talking about the illicit use of drugs, round which whole umbras and penumbras of sub-societies revolve, to ask what are the specific effects of this or that drug. Drugs are used quite differently in different social situations; very often the situation and the expectations of the user have far more effect than the chemical. Beer drunk in a rugger

	Craving	Pro-nounced psychic effects on adminis-tration	Psychic depen-dence	Toler-ance	Physical depen-dence	Psycho-toxic on with-drawal
Heroin and morphine	x		x	x	x	
Barbiturates	x	x	x	x	x	x
Alcohol	x	x	x	x	x	x
Bromides		x	x			x
Cocaine	x	x	x			
LSD		x	x	0		
Amphetamines	x	x	x			
Marihuana		x	x			
Nicotine	x		x			
Caffeine			x			x
Trousers			x		x	x

x means that major effects are often found, not that they always occur. Amphetamines are stimulants – methedrine, benzedrine, purple hearts, etc. 'Craving' means an immediate physical hunger. The 0 for LSD tolerance means that this drug is *anti*-addictive; after a few days' continuous use the effects vanish and cannot be re-established even by massive doses. It is worth noticing that only heroin, caffeine, nicotine and trousers produce no major psychic effects when they are taken. Trousers are included as another example of the similarity between drug-oriented behaviour and other relationships that we consider perfectly normal. We depend quite intensely on this substance, both mentally and physically, its withdrawal causes discomfort, mental distress, and is a well-known weapon in brain-washing.[3]

club is an excuse for taking trousers off; whisky in a pub in the Gorbals excuses hitting your friends with bottles; Bloody Marys at a Chelsea party facilitate sexual advances towards other people's wives. Each society uses alcohol as a key to unlock different forms of behaviour – activities one would never guess at from the controlled administration of the drug in a laboratory.

Judged impartially alcohol is probably more harmful than heroin, because its prolonged use in itself causes physical and nervous deterioration, which heroin does not. If alcohol, instead of being a beneficent gift from the gods in the remote past, were invented today by a research chemist, there is little doubt it would immediately be stringently controlled by law. But because our society has lived with it so long, we can control it, and tolerate those effects we can't control. For example, it is estimated that there are about 100,000 acute alcoholics in England and Wales, and the upkeep of those that are in prison or who cannot work, with their families, costs the nation about £6 million a year. Less acute alcoholics are probably forty times as numerous, and their absenteeism and poor work costs, at a moderate estimate, another £35 million a year.[4] Seven to eight per cent of alcoholics eventually commit suicide.[9] Alcohol probably causes some 1,200 deaths on the roads and 50,000 injuries a year.[5] In Scotland alcoholism is the cause of admission to mental hospital of one patient in five. In Glasgow 15,000 crimes a year are committed under the influence of this drug, and in the three worst wards of the city six per cent of all males are arrested every year for being drunk and incapable.[6] These things happen around us and we are not worried. Our society spends £20 million a year advertising alcohol on TV and in the press,[7] and 340,000 people work at the manufacture and distribution of alcohol – half as many again as work in all gas, electricity and water supply industries.[8]

An alarming feature of the affluent society, even under economic pressure, is the increase in juvenile drunkenness. Between 1966 and 1973 there was a 36 per cent increase in prosecutions in England and Wales for under-age drinking. There was a threefold increase in admissions to mental hospitals for alcoholism in patients under 25. The teenage violent alcoholic emerged as a challenge to discipline in schools – an educational problem hitherto unknown.[10] This pattern is not peculiar to the United Kingdom, but has been noted with justifiable alarm in many countries of the West, particularly America, Canada, Germany and Scandinavia. In terms of numbers affected, it probably far outweighs any other drug, but because government revenues everywhere depend on substantial income from taxation on the sale of alcohol, little is likely to be done about it.

Alcohol for us is a useful and necessary part of life. In other contexts it has been socially catastrophic, decimating populations and destroying cultures. Its impact on unsophisticated people who had not developed our complex of social controls was a powerful weapon in the last century's spread of European civilization in America, Australia, Africa. In the same way, the culture that goes with a drug is as important as the pharmacology of the stuff. Cannabis was, and is, used in the Far East to assist meditation and religious out-of-self-ness; the assassins or Haschischiens took it to make them ferocious; in Cairo in the thirties it was the centre of a nationalist, anti-British movement; American jazz musicians use it socially, and feel it improves their musical sensitivity; students here take it as an emblem of rebellion. In each situation the drug induces different effects. So we must also look at the people who use these problem drugs, and the circumstances in which their use meets with approval from others.

Since heroin and the opiates are the archetypal drugs of addiction – that is, if it were not for them, we would hardly be so conscious of drug problems – the next three chapters are devoted to them. In the next chapter we examine what is known of the drugs' pharmacology and the clinical behaviour of users; Chapter 3 deals with the addict's psychology, and Chapter 4 with the myths that he and society weave around drugs.

2
Archetypal Heroin

The Beginnings of Dependence

Although the number of heroin users in this country is statistically negligible – estimates vary between totals of 400 and 2,000, or between 0·8 and 4 per hundred thousand of the population – this is the archetypal drug of addiction, and round it we form our attitudes towards drugs and drug use generally.

Fifteen years ago Britain hardly had a drug problem, and had not had one since the turn of the century and the end of Victorian proprietary medicines that relied on opium for their remarkable cure-all effects. The Interdepartmental Committee on Drug Addiction (the Brain Committee) reported in this sense in 1961 : '. . . on the evidence before us the incidence of addiction to dangerous drugs was very small . . . there seemed no reason to think that any increase was occurring . . .'[1]

At that time, and for many years before, the addict population was a small, self-contained group of between three hundred and four hundred of whom about one in ten used heroin; most of these were elderly people who had contracted the habit through medical treatment. There were also about seventy doctors and nurses who had access to drugs and had probably started using them in some long period of duty when they also felt unusually ill and tired. There were a very small number of non-medical addicts – perhaps only a dozen. Richard H. is an example of one who has made an adequate adjustment to life. He is about forty-five, a thin, rather worried-looking man who worked for many years as the head of a design team in an advertising agency. His cuffs and collars are often frayed and sometimes a bit grimy; he is a bachelor and lives with a boyfriend and housekeeper in a neat little house by the river. His job brings him into emotional collision with a variety of people; he does his best to avoid arguments, which cause him almost physical pain. He is worried about

17

his job, about rivals in other firms, about his superiors and his subordinates. He treats everyone with the greatest politeness; yet intrigues incessantly. At lunch time he slips out to place disastrous bets; everyone likes him and sympathizes with the strain he suffers. He criticizes all about him with the most undiplomatic freedom.

He was young and at art school with several people who now have international reputations; then, just after they had begun their professional lives, he was the most successful. Now he is shy about them. Almost deliberately, it seems, he refuses to adjust to the rapidly changing modes of visual presentation. His work became old-fashioned in 1963 and he left his job. No one would have dreamed of asking him if he were an addict, and he certainly never talked about it.

He, and others like him, used heroin as a private, shameful accessory to their lives, for its pharmacological properties alone: to relieve anxiety, and to prevent withdrawal. That people can use opiates for twenty years or more without showing intellectual or moral deterioration is a common experience.

We think it must be accepted that a man is mentally or morally normal who graduates in medicine, marries and raises a family of useful children, practises medicine for 30 or 40 years, never becomes involved in questionable transactions, takes a part in the affairs of the community and is looked on as one of its leading citizens. . . . Such cases . . ., and they are not uncommon, have taken as much as 15 grains of morphine daily for years without losing one day's work because of morphine. Such addicts however are under the necessity of concealing a practice which is disapproved of by the public and proscribed by law. To this demoralizing situation is added the shame most of them feel at being the slave of a habit from which most of them would like to be free. This combination of furtive concealment and shameful regret cannot help but bring about some change for the worse in any personality, but the change produced in mature individuals is usually so slight that it cannot be demonstrated or cannot be classed as 'moral deterioration'.[2]

To these heroin plays much the same role as insulin to the diabetic, and they are by no means rare among people dependent on opiates. A more modern example from New England: a doctor who had a wife, a mistress, two children and a busy practice injected about a grain of morphine a day intramuscularly: 'one shot for patients, one for mistress, one for family, one to sleep'. When the mistress broke off the affair he went to a psychiatrist complaining of depression, but as soon as he could organize another mistress felt perfectly happy and went on as before.[3] This case also illustrates how drug dependence always accompanies other serious, social and psychological symptoms, and often appears to be the least that is wrong with the addict.

The New Addicts

But before the first report of the Brain Committee had been set up in type, the situation had changed so obviously that it could not be ignored. Instead of being passive, secretive people, addicts became publicists and proselytizers. Something like the American pattern of addiction began to emerge, with new addicts being actively recruited, mainly from adolescents, both working and middle class. Just how this self-perpetuating social pattern began is not at all clear. Looking back, the first sign of it was the arrest of a young professional trafficker in 1951 who had stolen a large amount of heroin and cocaine from a hospital pharmacy. In the three months he was at large in the West End of London he had built up a clientele of fifty customers. All of these, over the years, have emerged as confirmed addicts, who presumably have to some extent carried on their patron's energetic business habits.

An early contribution may have been made by the flight of addicts from Canada's new penal drug code of 1958. The first arrived at the end of 1959, and by the end of 1962 about 70 had come, some with criminal, trafficking backgrounds. By the end of 1965 about half had either died, returned voluntarily or been deported to Canada. We must also take into account the general change in teenage attitudes at the end of the fifties, with the shift of interest away from the crude external power relationships of gangs to rather more private worlds of experience expressed in clothes and music. In this changed atmosphere drug use might well be more readily accepted.[5]

Bewley gave an analysis of the number of heroin addicts known

19

to the Home Office, and their recruits, deaths, cures and deportations in each year from 1955 to 1964.[4] He reported that the number of new addicts each year followed a smoothly increasing curve, doubling roughly every nineteen months. A follow-up paper by the same author[30] carries the study forward to the end of 1966. He found the rate of increase slightly accelerated: the number of new cases reported doubled every sixteen months, and the total was 1,272. He predicted that there would be 800 new cases reported in 1967 and 1,200 in 1968. If the more or less stationary pre-1958 total of 60 addicts is subtracted from the yearly totals, it seems that every three 'new pattern' addicts recruited two more each year. But it became apparent that the totals of heroin addicts known to the Home Office (before the introduction of Treatment Centres and the registration of users) fell far short of reality. Just how far short was not apparent until Rathod and de Alarcón published their penetrating study[31] of teenage heroin users in Crawley New Town (one of the characterless new communities near London) over the years 1966–7. They found 27·21 known, probable or suspected heroin users per 1,000 among boys from 15 to 20. Their total, which may be incomplete, came to 92: a figure that contrasted strikingly with the eight cases there that had been reported by their doctors to the Home Office.

With a sudden rush of new young addicts, the Brain Committee was reconvened in 1964; its proposals and the chances of effective control of the situation are considered in Chapters 10 and 11. What it ignored, however, was one important aspect of the new wave: the favourable, indeed grasping, attitude to publicity of many young drug users.

This new brand of user makes addiction in itself a way of life, to be seen and commented on. Their drug dependence is an inarticulate but forceful statement about themselves and society; now that the subject of sex is being assimilated, this is perhaps the most shocking statement an adolescent can make. It is difficult to understand the spread of addiction unless one bears this in mind. The mythology and way of life of the heroin user plays as much part in the whole phenomenon as the pharmacology of the drug itself. We examine the myths in Chapter 4; here it is necessary to set out the salient facts about the drug.

The vital function of heroin, or any of the opiates whether natural or synthetic, seems to be their capacity for blotting out anxiety, and releasing the counter forces of confidence and euphoria. These drugs are used medically as painkillers, and although they dull the perception of pain, their more important function is to suppress the patient's alarm about the pain he still feels. A set of experiments at Lexington, the American hospital in Kentucky for the investigation and treatment of addiction, shows this rather neatly. Two experiments were set up, in both of which patients were asked to guess whether each of a series of shocks was more or less painful than a control shock. In one situation the experimenter treated the subjects amiably, there was no formality, and they could press the key to give themselves the shocks: most people graded them correctly. In the other set-up things were made very formal, everything was done in a curt and worrying way, and the actual electrical contact was made out of the patients' sight and without warning. In general these shocks were thought to be more painful than they actually were. Both sets were repeated with the subjects full of morphine. This time, apparently because worry over the second experimental situation was relieved by the drug, the subjects did as well as in the informal set-up.[6]

A more commonly given reason for addiction, which accords with the generally held mythology of drugs, is the 'kick', the sensuous pleasure on injection, particularly that produced by heroin. Opinions vary enormously about this. In some reports it is a sensation so poignant that no one can resist it. Nyswander says that some staff members at Lexington learned to feel the kick, and experienced it as a sort of orgasm in the stomach. She describes an addict getting his pay-off for helping in an experiment there: he chose to have a quarter grain of morphine injected into a neck vein.

There was a slow flush over his body; he rubbed his neck and his arms in an expression of pure joy and said: 'This is why men go to prison, and it's worth it' ... It is possible that the intensity of pleasure exceeds any pleasure known to non-addicts.[7]

21

She remarks in another passage that when long-term ex-addict prisoners, after three or four years' confinement, are asked whether they would like a luscious girl or a shot of morphine, they always say they would choose the drug. What are we to make of this evidence? It is possible they never particularly liked girls. Drug use often seems to correlate with inability to cope with the opposite sex. Then one must bear in mind that they have presumably been to, or heard about Lexington, where experiments are paid for in drugs. They might, by making contrary statements, hope to provoke an amusing trial of the matter.

Psychiatrists with a Freudian training often report that opiates are used as sex-substitutes.

Over and over again one hears addicts describe the effects of their injection in sexual terms. One addict said that after a fix he felt as if he were coming from every pore. Another said that he used to inject the solution in a rhythmic fashion until it was all used up, and said that this was akin to masturbation albeit much better.[8]

Many people feel no more than a warmth in the stomach and a tickling sensation in the crutch; the pleasure of this is often offset by the characteristic vomiting that the first shots of heroin or morphine produce. One ex-addict says that for a while 'it felt as though you had golden fire running through your veins', but this wore off, and towards the end of his self-terminated addiction he found heroin merely stupefying. Dr Goulding, one of the Secretaries of the Brain Committee, found that heroin had no more effect on him than a 'second-rate sleeping pill'. An experiment in which two successive doses of morphine were given to 150 healthy young men, found only three who would willingly allow the injection to be repeated, and none who would have sought it out. The authors conclude:

Opiates are not inherently attractive, euphoric or stimulant. The danger of addiction to opiates resides in the person and not the drug.[9]

From an earlier, classic paper on addiction:

The intensity of pleasure produced by opiates is in direct proportion to the degree of psychopathy of the person who becomes an addict....

The subsequent depression resulting from long continued use of the drug carries him as far below his normal emotional plane as his initial exaltation carried him above it.[10]

In other words perhaps: if one is emotionally very screwed up, relaxation feels marvellous, just as women feel positive sensations of pleasure when they take off tight shoes. But if one is relaxed to begin with the drug has no pleasure to offer.

The third important effect, which tends to continue drug use, is in no dispute: withdrawal. It is happily difficult to see this display of symptoms in Britain today, since addicts in prisons and hospitals are generally let down slowly under substitute opiates, tranquillizers and sedatives, but the fear of it is always in the addict's mind. It is indeed a spectacular and well documented medical drama. Dr Robert de Ropp describes it well:

'Withdrawal sickness' in one with well-developed physical dependence on opiates is a shattering experience and even a physician accustomed to the sight of suffering finds it an ordeal to watch the agonies of patients in this condition. About twelve hours after the last dose of morphine or heroin the addict begins to grow uneasy. A sense of weakness overcomes him, he yawns, shivers, and sweats all at the same time while a watery discharge pours from the eyes and inside the nose which he compares to 'hot water running up into the mouth'. For a few hours he falls into an abnormal tossing, restless sleep known among addicts as the 'yen sleep'. On awakening, eighteen to twenty-four hours after his last dose of the drug, the addict begins to enter the lower depths of his personal hell. The yawning may be so violent as to dislocate the jaw, watery mucus pours from the nose and copious tears from the eyes. The pupils are widely dilated, the hair on the skin stands up and the skin itself is cold and shows that typical gooseflesh which in the parlance of the addict is called 'cold-turkey', a name also applied to the treatment of addiction by means of abrupt withdrawal.

Now to add further to the addict's miseries his bowels begin to act with fantastic violence; great waves of contraction pass over the walls of the stomach, causing explosive vomiting, the vomit being frequently stained with blood. So extreme are the contractions of the intestines that the surface of the abdomen appears corrugated and knotted as if a tangle of snakes were fighting beneath the skin. The abdominal pain is severe and rapidly increases. Constant purging takes place and as many as sixty large watery stools may be passed in a day.

Thirty-six hours after his last dose of the drug the addict presents a truly dreadful spectacle. In a desperate effort to gain comfort from the chills that rack his body he covers himself with every blanket he can find. His whole body is shaken by twitchings and his feet kick involuntarily, the origin of the addict's term, 'kicking the habit'.

Throughout this period of the withdrawal the unfortunate addict obtains neither sleep nor rest. His painful muscular cramps keep him ceaselessly tossing on his bed. Now he rises and walks about. Now he lies down on the floor. Unless he is an exceptionally stoical individual (few addicts are, for stoics do not normally indulge in opiates) he fills the air with cries of misery. The quantity of water secretion from eyes and nose is enormous, the amount of fluid expelled from stomach and intestines unbelievable. Profuse sweating alone is enough to keep both bedding and mattress soaked. Filthy, unshaven, dishevelled, befouled with his own vomit and faeces, the addict at this stage presents an almost subhuman appearance. As he neither eats nor drinks he rapidly becomes emaciated and may lose as much as ten pounds in twenty-four hours. His weakness may become so great that he literally cannot raise his head. No wonder many physicians fear for the very lives of their patients at this stage and give them an injection of the drug which almost at once removes the dreadful symptoms. 'It is a dramatic experience,' writes Dr Harris Isbell, 'to observe a miserably ill person receive an intravenous injection of morphine, and to see him thirty minutes later shaved, clean, laughing and joking.' But this holiday from hell is of short duration and unless the drug is administered again all the symptoms start afresh within eight to twelve hours.* If no additional drug is given the symptoms begin to subside of themselves by the sixth or seventh day, but the patient is left desperately weak, nervous, restless, and often suffers from stubborn colitis.[11]

The tender de Ropp does not mention that both men and women suffer constant orgasms during the critical period.

The next effect, once physical dependence has been established, is the hunger of the addict for his drug when the amount of it circulating in his bloodstream falls below a comfortable point.

* These symptoms relate to morphine or heroin. It should be emphasized that synthetic drugs having a morphine-like action, such as pethidine, also give rise to addiction. The withdrawal symptoms are somewhat different. Addiction to pethidine is particularly common among doctors and nurses and is, according to Isbell, more harmful in its effects than addiction to morphine.

Just what happens inside the addict's body is uncertain – some lines of research are sketched below – but he feels the anxiety, irritability, discomfort of someone with powerful appetites who badly needs a meal, multiplied a hundred times. This appears to be a self-contained symptom, and not just a conscious attempt to avoid the withdrawal syndrome. The extremities of cunning and self-immolation this forces on addicts are well illustrated in this account:

I once treated a twenty-seven-year-old nurse, who complained of a recurrent cystitis, for which she had previously consulted one of my colleagues whose name she had obtained from a training hospital. She told him that she had had a kidney removed; a large scar on her back bore witness to this fact. She appeared to be in acute distress, with temperature, pallor, tenderness in the lumbar region. The physician did a urinalysis in his office and discovered crenated red blood cells which, together with other findings revealed in a thorough examination, seemed to substantiate her story. She stated that she was working as a nurse, and as she seemed to be quite intelligent, there was no reason for the physician to suspect anything out of the way.

She requested morphine but instead was given a prescription for Demerol, which she said she could administer herself. She phoned the next day to say that she was allergic to Demerol and asked him to leave a prescription for Dilaudid at the drugstore. He did so, and within twenty-four hours he called her to check on the condition. To his surprise, there was no such telephone number as the one she had given. When she again phoned for medication, the physician suggested that she first come in for another examination and mentioned the desirability of hospitalization. She made some excuse and he never heard from her again. He then realized that she was probably an addict, but he was puzzled about the appearance of crenated red blood cells in the urine.

Several months later this woman was arrested for stealing drugs from a hospital. She was sent to a prison-hospital and, by coincidence, I recognized her from my colleague's description of the diagnostic picture and her clever ruses to obtain drugs. A little probing cleared up the mystery of the crenated red blood cells: before she consulted a physician she put a small pencil up into her uretha, causing bleeding into the bladder.

This woman's entire period of hospitalization was characterized by self-inflicted injuries in an effort to obtain drugs while surgical repairs were being made. She swallowed, among other things, a wrist-watch, glass, broken pieces of silverware, stones and safety pins. In a continuous state of anxiety when off drugs, she could not work consistently. One night I was summoned to her room and found her sweating profusely, with dilated pupils and a low-grade temperature. She complained of a severe pain in her lumbar region. Examination of the urine showed crenated red blood cells. Despite the patient's previous history of feigning a kidney condition, she was given the benefit of the doubt and Demerol was prescribed until a medical work-up could be completed.

She continued to complain of severe pain and on the following day a flat plate of the abdomen revealed an opaque area in the region of the left ureter. On a tip from the technician, I examined the patient before she had her next X-ray and found on her back a flat wad of chewing gum mixed with some calcium-like material which would simulate a stone on the X-ray plate. The Demerol was stopped, but she continued to require medication from time to time and, in fact, demanded as much attention as ten other patients.

There was no doubt about this woman's difficult medical history and even in a purely custodial arrangement she could not cope with her problems. As a matter of fact, she hanged herself while doing a short term in a house of detention where she was forcibly and suddenly withdrawn from drugs. In my opinion, this particular patient needed drugs to handle her emotional and psychic turmoil just as the diabetic needs insulin in order to function well. Fortunately this type of case is a rarity.[12]

In time the kick weakens, the high vanishes, with good management withdrawal need never be experienced, and all the heroin addict has left is constant drowsiness, constipation, impotence, and the need for a slowly mounting dose.

The Pharmacology of Opiates

A considerable amount of work has been done on the internal action of drugs – much of it, one must admit, unintelligible to the layman – but there is no certainty yet on the mechanisms of their operation. One obvious fact is the power of opiates. The ordinary addict's dose of half a grain is roughly equivalent to only four millionths of the body's weight. On injection, heroin is immediately broken down into morphine and by-products. The lungs, liver and kidneys collect morphine readily, and soon after injection they contain a higher concentration than the blood. In fact, it is estimated that only between 2 per cent and 14 per cent is available as molecules free to enter brain tissue. An hour after rats were injected with two millionths of a gramme of morphine per gramme of body weight (equivalent to a dose of 2·4 grains for a well grown man) their brains contained no more than 0·09 millionths of a gramme per gramme of tissue, or 2 per cent of the concentration one would expect if the drug was distributed evenly through the body. The kidneys, on the other hand, contained 8,000 per cent of their share.[13]

This sort of evidence suggests that the effects of opiates may be due not so much to the drug, but to a body chemical released or inhibited by it. But the extreme difficulty of saying anything definite about the pharmacological action of drugs is illustrated by the work of Hill, who found that morphine – classically considered a depressant – could either slow down simple reaction times *or* speed them up, and that this effect depended solely on whether his subjects were paid for their cooperation *before or after* the experiment.[14]

In other experiments it is found that morphine both depresses and excites nervous activity. In cats with severed spinal cords habituation to opiates depresses one set of leg reflexes, and excites another pair; withdrawal spectacularly reverses these effects. One explanation of these phenomena is that morphine is absorbed quickly on the outer layers of nerve cells, giving a short-term stimulant effect, and slowly on the inside, producing habituation and depression. Another explanation points simply to the complex pyramidal nature of nervous organization; because of the function of some nerve cells in both exciting and inhibiting others, a single effect from the drug might be expected to produce widely different effects on the total organism. In the same way one might suppose that the drunkenness of a general might have effects on the behaviour of an army very different to the drunkenness of all the privates.

A more sophisticated idea is that morphine works by filling up keyhole-like positions on nerve cells that are normally occupied by molecules of a chemical called 5-hydroxytryptamine. In

27

reaction to this, the nerve cells develop more sites which are in turn slowly filled up by morphine molecules. While this slow invasion is going on, there is also a rapid metabolization of morphine molecules making it necessary for the addict to keep injecting the drug to keep up the coverage. Thus if there is enough morphine in the bloodstream things are functionally as normal: although there are far more receptor sites on the nerve cells most of them are covered up and no more 5-HT comes in contact with the nerves than necessary. But the growth of new receptor sites is always a jump ahead of the quantity of morphine present so the addict is slowly forced to step up his dose. After the last dose at the beginning of withdrawal the morphine is destroyed and not replaced, leaving the nerve cells over-supplied with receptor sites, and overwhelmed with 5-HT, which produces the well-known effects of withdrawal. In support of this idea, it is noticed that 5-HT is continuously produced in the brain, and that the effect of raising the 5-HT level in dogs closely resembles withdrawal. However, similar theories involving adrenaline, noradrenaline and other chemicals have been proposed.[15]

This general type of theory accounts for the interesting fact that withdrawal symptoms are opposite to the effects of the drug. It is suggested that the complex of signs felt during withdrawal – muscular pain, inability to keep still, air hunger, gooseflesh, nausea, bowel urgency, anxiety and the rest – are part of a deep-seated defence reflex which warns the body and prepares it for danger. The addiction-prone person is plagued by unwelcome sensations – which most of us feel only in the dentist's waiting-room – and takes the drug to be free of them. The euphoria he feels, and only he feels, is due to the relief of this pressure. On withdrawal he gets back, very literally, the accumulated reflex that he has avoided during addiction.[16]

Intermediate between the involuntary autonomic nervous effects of opiates and their withdrawal, and the conscious elements of the addict's life, lies the craving for the drug, and the compulsion to obtain it. The plaintiveness and ingenuity of addicts' attempts to get opiates are very characteristic. One example was described on p. 25; every doctor who treats addicts can describe similar cases of this personality aberration. Animals show the same behaviour. In one experiment a group of chimpanzees was trained to solve problems for food rewards. Naturally enough they were then hardly interested by the offer of a syringe of morphine; after addiction their performance for food was low, but for the syringe high.[17]

An unusually brutal experiment in America shows the importance of the fore-brain in craving. Four patients who were about to have bilateral frontal lobotomies – three for schizophrenia, and one for phantom limb pain – were addicted and withdrawn. Whether this was done with the patients' permission is not stated. Disappointingly the schizophrenics showed all the involuntary signs of withdrawal, but did not make the characteristic faces and demands of the normal addicts. The fourth man responded in the usual way, asking repeatedly and pathetically for a dose of morphine. After one-sided lobotomy had been done on all four the process was repeated with the same result; again the phantom limb man was the only one to show craving. After the second lobotomy none of them showed any but the non-purposive signs of withdrawal – vomiting, gooseflesh, loss of weight and so on.[6]

This section was intended as no more than a rough guide to the sort of ideas that are being investigated in this difficult field. So far, it is safe to say, theoretical investigations of opiate addiction have thrown some useful light on the working of the nervous system, but hardly contributed yet to solutions of the problems caused by these drugs.

Addiction in Britain

Heroin addiction has now been a social problem in Britain long enough for some research to have been done on it, and for some facts to emerge. A survey of heroin users in some, unnamed, industrial town, taken in 1967 and repeated in 1968,[32] found that of fifty heroin users, 84 per cent were male, and their average age was 21 – that of the girls 19, and almost all were single. Social classes I and II were over-represented and Class V underrepresented. Half of them took heroin daily, and their dosage ranged from $\frac{1}{8}$ of a grain to 5 grains. Among the other half, 36 per cent used the drug irregularly, 4 per cent were in hospitals or prisons, and 12 per cent had given it up.

The national statistics on addiction, as published by the Home Office,[33] show a remarkably high turnover, with, recently, a fall in the number of known addicts. Thus, of 2,782 known addicts during 1968, 61 died, and 965 dropped out. In 1969, 64 died, 1,351 dropped out, and 1,135 started, leaving, at the end of the year, 1,466 users of heroin and methadone.

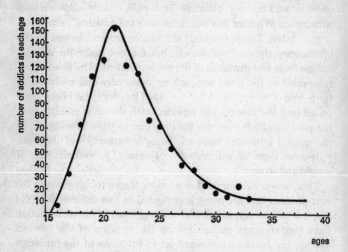

Figure 1. This graph shows the numbers of known British heroin and methadone users plotted against their age. The great majority are in their early twenties. Source, reference 33.

American Addiction

Opiate addiction has, until recently, been such a rarity in Britain that it has hardly been worth investigating it. America, on the other hand, has devoted enormous resources to the investigation and treatment of this condition. The material on addiction is therefore largely due to American workers. The dependence of addiction on culture and the expectations of the addict is so important that one can only offer this as suggestive material; but the similarity between Britain and America is enough for us to see the relevance of many American findings to our own problems.

American investigators have the advantage of two State hospitals – Lexington, Kentucky, opened 1935, and Fort Worth, Texas, opened 1938, which treat both voluntary and convict addicts. There is a Federal Bureau of Narcotics, curiously enough under the control of the Treasury, which keeps records of active addicts, and claims that no one can use drugs illicitly for more than two years without being recorded. Addiction is spread over America in an interesting way. Broadly one can say that it occurs where the opportunity to get drugs co-exists with social and economic squalor. An analysis of the admissions to the two hospitals shows two main patterns.[18] The 'southern' pattern, a survival from 1915, is found in Alabama, Georgia, Kentucky. Addicts tend to be 90 per cent white, aged about 43, and usually using the old morphine mixtures: pergoric, Dilaudid, and sometimes morphine itself. The modern pattern of imported heroin use is found in New York, Puerto Rico, the District of Columbia and Chicago. Two thirds of those from the first three States are Negro or Puerto Rican, and their average age is about 27. A narrow belt of heroin use is growing near the borders with Mexico in Arizona, New Mexico and Texas. Both these patterns continue phenomena described in 1928 by Kolb[19] and by Terry and Pellens.[20] It is also possible to compare Lexington's population now with that in 1937, when the first study of the hospital's intake was made.[21] In 1937 the southern type was more common and outweighed admissions from New York and Illinois. During the interruption of world communications during the Second World War heroin was very difficult to come by and addiction rates fell. After the war it rose again to a peak of 1,823 cases in 1950, and is now slowly falling.[18] This drop, and the distribution of Lexington and Fort Worth compulsory admissions, correlates well with the Federal Bureau of Narcotics' file, but Ball and Cottrell comment that unfortunately this file is probably not a reliable guide to the total number of addicts, since there is little demographic relationship between the voluntary patients – who make up about a third of the Lexington population,

31

and four fifths of the admissions[22] – and the Bureau's records.[23] Obviously the underprivileged addict who lives in a criminal, addict society has a far better chance of being picked up than, say, a respectable doctor living in a small town in the centre of the country.

In twenty-five years the mean age of addicts has fallen by eight years to 33·5. In 1937 less than one male patient in five was under 30, in 1962 almost half were. Before the war 10 per cent of the patients were non-white; now one third are Negro, 12 per cent Puerto Rican, 5 per cent Mexican. An examination of young addicts admitted to a New York hospital, ingeniously controlled against their non-addict friends, showed the joint importance of social as well as psychiatric reasons for addiction in this group. The authors comment that urban Negroes and Puerto Ricans have very low status and very high rates of hospitalization for all mental illnesses, especially dementia praecox (schizophrenia). They are particularly susceptible to alcohol psychoses, delinquency and TB. Curiously, the addicts often seemed to come from homes that outwardly seemed better than average, but it often turned out that the parents had unrealistic attitudes towards life, or simply denied the difficulties of life in the slums. In these homes the parents were more concerned with status – new furniture, a big car outside – than with security or the advancement of their children through education and work. The authors conclude that 'addicts exceeded the controls in personality malfunction to a statistically significant and clinically impressive extent . . . youths . . . do not become addicted independent of psycho-pathology'.[24]

Ball comments that 'there has been a notable increase in the number of addicts from the minority groups in American society'.[25] We in Britain are less likely to be faced with the problems of ghettoes on the Harlem scale, but we should not be complacent about the safety of our own second or third generation coloured immigrant populations. Cultural underprivilege is not something static: advance in one part of society generates deprivation in another. Our own addicts seem to come not from distinct ethnic underprivileged groups, but more from an underprivileged class: the teenagers, who are both exposed to and denied many of the pleasures and opportunities of our own society.

The Myths of Inevitable Addiction and the Pusher

Although it is possible to demonstrate some physical adaptation even to one day's use of heroin, by injecting the antidote nalorphine which precipitates an immediate withdrawal, it takes something like half a grain a day for a fortnight before anyone is even mildly physically dependent on the drug.[19] Even then the withdrawal will be nothing worse than a mild dose of flu, lasting a couple of days. The idea of instant addiction after one dose is not substantiated. Addiction must, in fact, be the result of continued, conscious action, with some deterrents to be overcome like vomiting, the unpleasantness of sticking needles into veins, the expense and trouble of buying the drug on the black market. Add to this the later 'sitting round in doctors' waiting rooms, having to find somewhere to shoot up, feeling sick before a shot, feeling sick after it and then sleepy'. 'It all became a bore. You have to work at being an addict,' says one who gave it up.

This impression is confirmed by Chein's study for the New York Youth Board of New York adolescent drug users. He and his associates found that in the most desolate 15 per cent of the city, where 75 per cent of the addicts live, although narcotics of a sort were available on every street corner, only one boy in ten tried heroin over the four-year study period, and far fewer became addicted. There it is quite common for the kids to joy pop at weekends for years, without ever getting a large enough dose to produce withdrawal symptoms and force dependence on them.[9]

In America before the passage of the Harrison Act in 1914 one could buy opiates either raw or mixed in patent medicines at every pharmacy.* Yet of a population of 100 millions, it is estimated that only 100,000 were addicted. That is one per thousand

---

*The impact of opiates on nineteenth-century Americans is shown by an analysis of 10,000 prescriptions made up by Boston drugstores in 1888: altogether 1,481 contained opiates; so did 25% of those renewed once, 61% of those renewed twice and 78% of those renewed three times.[2]

at the beginning of the century; fifty years of vicious repression has reduced this to one per three thousand.

An extremely interesting contribution to the problem of addict recruitment was unwillingly made by the United States Army out of its experiences in Vietnam. There, no doubt with the energetic help of the Vietcong, some 30 per cent of its soldiers became addicted to heroin. It must be said that only 10 per cent injected it, while the rest smoked the drug, but nonetheless, they had genuine physical habits. As if this were not bad enough – for an addicted soldier is not the most aggressive fighting machine, and the logistic problem of supplying his habit must have been enormous – on return to the U.S.A. many of these men claimed disability pensions on the grounds that heroin addiction is permanent and disqualifies the sufferer from any sort of productive life. Apart from the expense of the pensions, the political repercussions of so many conscripts 'wounded' in such a way, which the American people have been taught to associate with the utmost depravity, would have been most damaging to the Army. So the military authorities were forced to embark on a research programme which followed up returned soldiers and found that – as one might expect – only 1 per cent[35] continued as addicts in the calmer conditions of their native land. One can well understand that the circumstances of fighting the war in Vietnam would in themselves be a very good reason for addiction in the most normal person, and once they were removed there would be no reason to continue.

It is also a fantasy that in a black market under conditions of repression addicts are made by the pressure and organized wiles of pushers and traffickers. An authoritative American handbook says:

The susceptible person does not, as a rule, start out looking for a shot and he is not, as a rule, coaxed into taking one by a 'pusher' for the illegal drug trade. Ordinarily he is introduced to drugs by his associates.[3]

The practice of handing out free or cheap samples at random in the hope of landing a customer is both uneconomic and dangerous

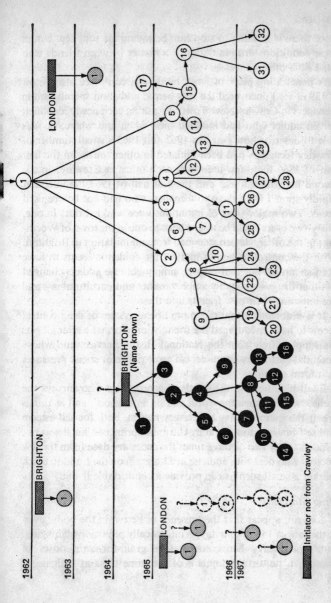

Figure 2. This diagram shows how heroin abuse spread in Crawley from four to six initial drug users to a total of fifty-eight by the end of 1967. (After de Alarcón)

since there is nothing to stop him betraying his supplier. Under these conditions drug initiation is a matter between friends who trust each other.

A penetrating piece of work by de Alarcón[34] (see also below p. 139 *et seq.*) uncovered the way heroin addiction spread among teenagers in Crawley New Town. By asking each newly identified heroin addict who had initiated him, when and where, he was able to describe how between 1962 and 1965 a small number of Crawley teenagers had been initiated in other towns. In the first half of 1966 these few users met each other in Crawley; in the second half of that year and the first half of 1967 the infection rapidly spread from them to teenagers who had not before used drugs. Two major trees of initiations were winkled out: in one, thirty-two users could be traced back to one in the town of Worthing; in the other, sixteen stemmed from an initiation in Brighton. With the control of heroin in 1968 the epidemic seems to have been stemmed, but that may be simply because addicts changed to other drugs – probably amphetamines and barbiturates – and are initiating their new friends into these.

It is unfortunate that our more liberal system of drug control seems to have encouraged the friendly initiator, who after all gets his supplies free from the National Health Service, and whose potential customers are under no great police or social pressures to inform on him.

English addicts, in the words of a prostitute who surveys the scene, 'want to turn the world and its mother on', and as things are at the moment they have every reason, both for self-esteem and self-interest, to keep at it. Until the spring of 1968 it was not difficult to get two or three times the necessary dose from the few doctors who deal with addicts; at £1 a grain on the London black market a small surplus can provide a comfortable living.

Drug Morbidity

It does not appear that the presence of heroin in the body, even at the rate of 15 grains a day, is intrinsically physically damaging. But most heavy heroin users take grain-for-grain doses of cocaine, a powerful stimulant of the same class as caffeine or amphetamine, to reduce the numbing effect of the opiate. It is possible that much of the harm attributed to heroin is in fact caused by cocaine hydrochloride. In medical practice cocaine, the oldest local anæsthetic, is considered too dangerous for injection, since it is an intense stimulant of the central nervous system. In large doses it causes acute paranoia, and in some cases 'a sudden, rapid and fatal collapse'.[25] Because of its powerful anaesthetic properties, the flesh it touches is unusually apt to suffer secondary damage: habitual cocaine sniffers tend to lose the partition between their nostrils. But large doses of heroin seem to produce fewer ill effects than large doses of alcohol, which cause peripheral neuritis – the deterioration of the long nerve cells joining the fingers and toes to the spinal column, producing tingling, insensitive, clumsy hands and feet. The major damage in both cases is done by the way of life that accompanies heavy drug use: irregular meals, insufficient vitamin intake, insanitary living; these overwhelmingly hurt health.

The medical complications commonly found among addicts at Lexington are: 'Serum hepatitis [a sort of jaundice], venereal diseases, malnutrition, skin infection with residual scars, superficial venous thrombosis [swelling and blocking of the arm veins used for injections], abscess formation both of the skin and internal organs, acute intoxication from accidental overdosage, amenorrhoea, fungus diseases of the skin, respiratory diseases [pneumonia, tuberculosis, bronchial asthma], psychosomatic disorders, peridontal disease and dental caries.'[26] This is confirmed among British addicts by Bewley,[30] who also finds that 60 per cent of British heroin addicts have some signs of liver damage.

The morbidity of opiate use is equally debatable. On the one hand there are the cases quoted at the beginning of this chapter who go on for decades, on the other adolescents who are dead after a couple of months. Since no one knows accurately either the number of addicts at risk, or the number who die, it is extremely difficult to come to any firm conclusions. O'Donnell followed up a large group of Kentucky addicts: over half had died in the twelve years since their first discharge from Lexington, of murder, suicide, disease, accidents, infections and mental illnesses.[28] On the other hand Winick's study of drop-outs from the Federal Bureau of Narcotics' active file showed a considerable number who had been addicted for thirty-five years or more, and one who had kept going for fifty-six years.[29]

In New York about 350 deaths a year occur among about 35,000 addicts.[27] In England, up to the end of 1966, there had been 69 deaths from 2,532 'addict years at risk', giving a mortality rate of 27 per 1,000 per year, nearly three times the New York rate and twenty-eight times the rate for non-addicts of similar ages. In 1968 and 1969 the rate fell slightly to 22 per 1,000.[33] But the calculation of morbidity depends as much on the numbers of drug users at risk as on the number of deaths. We only know the numbers of heroin and methadone users; there may be ten times as many people involved in the drug world, and equally at risk. The extremely high apparent death rate may also be because addicts often aren't identified until they die. But it is certain that, on average, addicts die sooner than non-addicts.

Perhaps what kills is not so much the drug as the personality that uses it self-destructively, that gives itself overdoses, that fails to take simple sanitary precautions with injections; that in fact wants to kill itself without having to make the decision to do so. It is not true simply to say that to become addicted is to embark on a slow, painful suicide.

One distinguished psychiatrist, who runs a hospital clinic, even sees heroin addiction as a welcome triumph of natural selection over the National Health Service. In his view addiction singles out weak people who would, in earlier times, have died before reaching maturity, and even if it doesn't kill them, it prevents them breeding – to the benefit of the race.

3
The Psychology of the Addict

The Personality of the Addict

A useful definition of the person who becomes dependent on drugs is given by Winick:

> The drug addict is a person with certain personality characteristics who happens to have selected this way of coping with his problems for a variety of reasons of which he is usually unaware. Not the least of these reasons is his access to a social group in which drug use was both practised and valued.[1]

This accounts neatly for the doctor, the therapeutic and the beatnik addict. But what sort of personality is susceptible; why does one person persevere after a shot while his friend does not? Why does one patient doped with heroin develop a craving while the man in the next bed does not? The key seems to be again in the opiates' power to obliterate worry.

Anxiety is the mental mechanism that forces action to satisfy the basic drives to find food, shelter, a mate. It is the pain that overcomes the sloth of the flesh. It is possible that there are people who, because of their mental make-up, of their up-bringing, or more probably both together, are over-driven; they are never unworried, and their lives are a constant pain to them. Every unkind word hurts, every difficulty seems insurmountable, every success trifling. Almost all accounts of people who are dependent on drugs stress that they have, continuously, a very bad opinion of themselves and their abilities. The addict never feels the occasional sunburst of self-satisfaction that encourages the rest of us to plug on with life. Most of us cope with anxiety by altering the situation that causes it. A young man, for example, settles his late-adolescent anxiety about his place in life by em-barking on a career; a course of action that may produce more immediate worries. But he is stable enough to take a long-term view; set-backs now are played off against long-term successes. But the addict cannot believe that anything which does not make him feel better *now* will ever make him feel better. Since few situations in life are open to immediate alteration, he prefers, or he is driven, to eliminate anxiety itself. For most of us it is a useful spur; for him a juggernaut. Since whenever a situation becomes painful he uses heroin to eliminate his drive to follow it through, it is not surprising he seldom has a job, or a home, or a wife. Here we have one powerful reason for opiate dependence; it is self-perpetuating in another way, for the more often anxiety is avoided, the less easy it is going to be to face it alone.

The action [of heroin and morphine] on the central nervous system is that the addict feels he has eaten to his heart's content, experienced full sexual satisfaction and eliminated all his anxieties as well. One begins to see that the behaviour of addicts is bound to be utterly different from that of people whose major drive centres round appeasing these basic life factors.[2]

One might also add that the addict misses the more intense pleasure got from the *process* of satisfying these drives; he has to be content merely with the feelings of satiation afterwards.

It is interesting to consider another question. Assuming that these people need something to modify their personalities, 'to take them out of themselves', why do they choose heroin, which is hard to get and brings social disapproval, rather than alcohol which is readily available? The pharmacological part of the answer lies in the diametrically opposite effects of the two drugs. Both deal with anxiety over sexuality and aggression: alcohol, by eliminating inhibition, enables one to act freely; heroin, by removing the drive, makes it unnecessary to act. It is suggested that people tend to use the drug that reinforces their method of handling these drives. In America, and to a lesser extent in Britain, where men are expected to be aggressive and adequately sexed, the majority use alcohol. (It is interesting that in parts of the East, where passivity is preferred, the approved drug is cannabis, another pacifier, and alcohol is held in the same horror as we hold heroin.)[3] In the West the minority use heroin to facilitate their naturally passive solution, and it may be that the disapproval this practice causes is aroused by its denial of the basic power source of Western social organization: the self-seeking drive of the male.

Inquiry into the personalities of American addicts tends to confirm this theory. (Unfortunately there has not been any similar study of English addicts.) Chein found that the typical adolescent addict in New York was a pretty, symmetrical, coloured boy; a dandy who would wear a goatee and try to behave like a gentleman. A boy, in short, who had completely opted out of the American Male ideal.[4] At the beginning of their inquiry the psychiatrists found themselves almost coming to blows over their descriptions of the boys' personalities. Each addict seemed a different person to each inquirer; they concluded that the addict's make-up was typically fluid and plastic, concealing an inward collection of negative characteristics: inability to have friendly relationships, difficulty with being masculine (probably more important in America than here, where teenagers tend towards outward monosexuality), feelings of futility, depression, being easily frustrated and made anxious and finding these feelings intolerable.

It seemed they often came from homes where the father was non-existent or failed to function, and where the mother was unusually dominant. Another study of mature addicts found more than a third still living with female relatives at the age of thirty – twice as many as one would expect in a prison population which was otherwise comparable.[5] Often these addicts' homes would seem to the casual caller to be better furnished and kept than the average. What the visitors could not see was a childhood spent as one of the furnishings of the home, an object to his parents, rather than a person in his own right.

Chein's study found that the personality problems of young addicts are just the same as those of the more mature – another blow at the 'pusher corrupting innocence' idea. It emerged that three things were necessary to form an addict: (1) a psychological, predisposing inadequacy; (2) a crisis; (3) the timely offer of drugs. The 'crisis' may be nothing in objective terms – perhaps only the problem of asking a girl to dance at a Saturday evening hop – but enough when it faces such a personality caught in the throes of adolescence. *Narcotic Drug Addiction* goes on to say:

> Youngsters who experiment with drugs know that what they are doing is both illicit and dangerous, but they have a delinquent attitude towards life. Eighth grade boys with a favourable attitude to the use of drugs view life with pessimism, unhappiness and a sense of futility, and they distrust authority.

> The chances of a boy's being exposed to drugs depends to a large extent on his being associated with delinquent groups. . . . The boy who eventually took drugs had no strong incentive to suppress impulse and develop discipline; since the father was absent, or cool, or hostile, the child had relatively little chance to model himself after a male figure; most of the parents had unrealistically low ambitions for their boys, reflecting their own pessimistic attitudes towards life, and they were distrustful of teachers, social workers and other representatives of society.[6]

With different phrasing, the same assessment sounds like abuse:

> Addicted patients are asocial, inadequate, immature and unstable. They are selfish and self-centred without any interest in the welfare of others and are only concerned in their own problems. Their major problem is in the maintenance of the supply of drugs or the immediate gratification of their desire for drugs. They will resort to any means – however unreasonable or dangerous – to satisfy this insistent craving. They have failed to develop normal human relationships and are almost totally without concern for the distress they inflict on their relatives. They lack self-discipline, will-power or ambition, and avoid responsibility. They have a low threshold for pain or any form of discomfort and are unable to tolerate criticism or to bear frustration. Their personal relationships tend to become confined to other members of the drug addicts' world and thus they become social outcasts and very lonely people.[7]

We have to make allowances in transferring the characteristics of American drug users to our own culture, but the pattern seems remarkably basic. This is not to say that one can predict with any certainty who will become dependent on drugs and who will not. The variables of opportunity and event are multiplied by the supreme variable of personality, but one can at least recognize the characteristics of the existing addict as readily here as in

America. Here, as an exercise in hindsight, is the story of Stephen North, an eighteen-year-old who lived in Pimlico.

His mother has a nice rebuilt flat in one of those bleak tenement blocks put up by charitable trusts at the turn of the century. She stood at the door in the dark hallway rubbing her eyes. She wore carpet slippers; she'd been dozing before the convector fire, waiting for her youngest son to come home from school. The winter afternoon light hardly reached through the lace curtain, so the smart black sofa and the woolly carpet glowed red from the heater. She says:

After he left school at fifteen he had trouble with purple hearts and pills. He used to go up these dance clubs in Soho – they should be blown up if you ask me. He was very unsettled and he didn't want to work; so they sent him on probation to a farm in Kent. He liked that really, and when he came home last spring he seemed much more settled. Well, he even went down to the Labour Exchange and got himself a job with an antique restorer's. He was ever so happy because he's always had artistic leanings. He joined the T.A. then, and he *was* looking forward to their trip to Germany in the summer.

Then, that weekend. Well, I've lived it over and over in my mind, he came home Friday very cheerful and went out with his girlfriend Jinnie. And again on Saturday. Only he didn't come home that night. Well, he's done that before, he stays over at her parents' place, so I didn't worry. In the morning before eight, there's Jinnie banging at the door. 'He's gone all blue,' she says, so I went round there straightaway. The night before he'd gone off to sleep on the sofa watching tele, so they covered him up and went to bed. In the morning they couldn't wake him, and he didn't look well, but the mother – silly woman – went off to work. Of course I called the ambulance, but he was dead.

They said at the inquest that it was bronchial pneumonia brought on by heroin. They said he'd been an addict for three weeks. Apparently he'd shared a pill with a boy on the estate and gone on from there. It doesn't seem long, does it? I never thought . . . It hurts when people say, 'You should have known.' How could I know? He didn't do nothing different. I didn't look him over for needle marks in the bath. If they'd got the ambulance straight away, he could have lived. They got the stuff from this Gypsy Curtis who used to hang about Piccadilly Circus selling cheap shots to kids – until he got them hooked. They arrested him the next day, and he died in Brixton the day after. Drowned in his own vomit when they stopped his drugs. He *was* a putrid character if you please.

Stephen's father? No comment. It's got to the stage where he goes out and gets drunk, and that's that. Stephen used to say, 'Don't you take no notice of him' – he was ever so nice to me. It used to upset him when he was younger, but now he'd got used to it. He was very soft-hearted; he hated to be called a chicken. He was always having accidents because people dared him to do stupid things. Perhaps that's why he took the tablet. He had his moods too – he'd either be up in the air, or down in the dumps. He was a very nice boy. Everybody said so.

The Psychological Function of Addiction

We have examined some personality characteristics that appear to cause people to *become* addicts if they get the opportunity; it is also interesting to identify the psychological mechanisms that *continue* addiction. The important thing is that 'his life adds up to a self-enclosed system where he is able to provide his own pleasure. . . . He isolates himself beyond the need for human help or satisfaction. He is dependent on no other person.'[2] His regularly recurring periods of euphoria are balanced by the equally frequent periods of come-down; it seems that the self-punishment of finding drugs as well as incipient withdrawal is as important in the addict's personal universe as the enjoyment of his high.

Scenes of laying in dank, funky, goddam hotel rooms. Sick as a dog. You know, too weak to care. You know, where literally you do not wash or dress. To go out, you try to stop your heaving long enough to put your clothes on. Forget about combing your hair, washing your face. It's ridiculous. Just put a cap over your head, and hope for the best. And there's moments when you really don't care. 'Get me some money, or go to the penitentiary' is the attitude [of the pusher]. You know, too weak. It's raining. Snowing. Freezing. And it's a Sunday morning, and you look out and there's loads of snow and your shoes got holes in them. All the clothes in the world won't keep you warm. And it's Sunday. And you don't got enough junk.[8]

Always preferring the short-term gratification to the long-term satisfaction, his continual victory over the withdrawal crisis – which is represented in junkie folklore as an unparalleled catastrophe:

'Man, it's like your skeleton's trying to jump outa your skin,' says a London seventeen-year-old – makes his way of life continually self-justifying. At the same time it disqualifies him, either because he's feeling too ill, or he is too busy looking for drugs, from attempting any other way of life that might lead to deeper satisfaction, but would also expose him to criticism and competition. He takes this course because he has the poorest opinion of himself; he knows he cannot compete on ordinary terms and feels he is doomed to a life of being inferior and despised. Drugs alone offer him a way out of this situation. Nyswander quotes the story of a boy who ran away from school and began a life of crime and addiction because his teacher laughed at his spelling. 'Drugs give him the satisfactions of the aggressor – over sexual repletion, etc. – while maintaining his passivity.'[2] Another view:

His conception of himself is that of a fairly worthless creature who can hardly move about in society without a constant barrage of anxiety. [With drugs] he leaves the world of symbolic interaction behind in one fundamental sense: for although he may continue to function as a medical practitioner, a musician, etc., he is no longer dependent on it for his sense of self-value.[9]

This continual stilling of anxiety with heroin very powerfully conditions him towards heroin use in difficult circumstances. Wikler suggests that this explains how a man can be cured of his addiction, live apparently successfully for fifteen years or so, then his business fails, or his wife leaves him, and he is back on the needle again. Even more curiously, one dose in a lapse of this sort will bring on a powerful withdrawal reaction, even when this is pharmacologically impossible. It seems that the whole chemical pattern of drug behaviour is reinforced by learning.[10] This has been strikingly confirmed by rat experiments. Wikler found that rats addicted to morphine and then withdrawn showed more withdrawal symptoms if they were kept in surroundings familiar to them during their addiction than if they were moved.[14] Another series of experiments showed that rats trained to give themselves injections of morphine when they felt withdrawal symptoms coming on, used more morphine when they got into difficulties and relapsed more easily than rats who were trained to use it simply for pleasure. [15, 16, 17]

Explanations of drug addiction in terms of an inadequate psyche or Pavlovian learning theory follow traditional paths of psychiatry. A more recent suggestion[18] sees addiction in terms of the addict's *operation*, and explains it as a reaction to an excess of leisure. The point of addiction then is to provide a rigid framework for the addict's life. On heroin, almost every minute of the day is prescribed: the user is either fixing, high, coming down, out boosting to buy more drugs, scoring, fixing again. His life goes in eight-hour cycles, and it is significant that the drug chosen has the shortest cycle period of any available opiate. It is put forward in support of this idea that heroin addicts are often model prisoners, because they welcome the discipline of prison, and that cures using coercion (p. 145) are far more successful than those without. In this view the present epidemic of heroin addiction is a reaction of inadequate personalities to a society in which people can eat without working, and in which there is nothing people *have* to do. A working-class Victorian boy, of the personality type that would now become an addict, would not have to use drugs because he would work from dawn to dark. He would have no agonizing decisions to make about what he should do, where he should be.

It is not easy to diagnose a long-standing heroin habit without chemical analysis of the urine, or provoking a withdrawal. Apart from the need to inject the drug, there may be no outward signs of dependence at all if the dose is nicely calculated to the addict's tolerance. He then behaves perfectly normally, though if one could compare him to his unaddicted self, he would show less nervous tension. Before addiction in itself was recognized, or became politically and morally unacceptable, opium was used at the end of the last century to calm vicious criminals without fogging their minds.[11] The real objection to long-term use of opiates is that the need for them becomes, to the addict, a primary one replacing the needs for sex or food, whose satisfaction serves no useful social purpose.

Wikler describes a most interesting, if rather cold-blooded, experiment in which an ex-addict was allowed to re-addict himself in the certainty that at a given time his supply of drugs would be cut off. The candidate was under psychiatric observation during the experiment, and himself chose the size and frequency of his doses entirely as he wished. The man selected had had a spectacular career as a speedboat driver during Prohibition. At the age of twenty-two he would drive his boat all night, get home in the early morning, sleep three or four hours and then smoke a pipe of opium. He would go out to a meal, then spend long afternoons and evenings smoking his pipe with a few friends.

He thought withdrawal from morphine unpleasant, but no deterrent, and readily agreed to the experiment. Normally he was rather guarded towards the hospital staff, but after his re-addiction had started he showed more hostility, and was full of stories of the guards being unfair to the other patients. By the end of five months he had raised his dose to nearly twelve shots of two grains a day, or a total of twenty-four grains (still a long way from the highest known dose of seventy-five grains). As the experiment proceeded, he welcomed his increased tolerance and craving, 'It's nice to be hooked, because when you're not it's like a good friend's gone away'; it meant that he could enjoy the thrill of injection more often: 'A steak tastes good at any time, but even better if you're hungry.' He would work two hours a day at filing, and spent the rest of his time lying on his bed, listening to the radio, dozing, and saying he wouldn't get hooked. A month before his supplies were stopped he was warned, and offered advice on tapering off and transferring to methadone. This he did for three weeks, but two days before the end he pushed his dose right back up again and suffered a spectacular withdrawal.

Although he had felt guilty during the experiment because he was becoming hooked again against his will, and because he was enjoying the luxury of opiates when his fellow prisoners could not, he felt all this had been expiated by his withdrawal. Although he had consumed the junkie's equivalent of a fortune of drugs, with very little outcome, since his projected analysis under morphine was largely abortive, he still demanded payment in opiates for help in further experiments. He obviously felt that withdrawal had discharged his debts; he owed no one any favours over that transaction. Wikler suggests that this need and ability to pay off one's guilt internally suggests why addicts so often choose heroin, the drug that hooks the hardest and from which one falls the furthest, although morphine, meperidine and methadone all produce euphoria. To the addict, the withdrawal or its threat is necessary counterbalance to the high; thus, in spite of his disesteem which prescribes guilt for every satisfaction, he is able to have his pleasure and live free of pain.[12]

Analysis of the addict personality generally takes the form of enumerating externally apparent characteristics. There is little attempt to *understand* why he behaves as he does, partly perhaps because such a projection into such a different way of behaviour is difficult even for a trained psychiatrist, partly perhaps because if we understand we can hardly condemn. The closer we get to the centre of the problem, the closer we come to the dilemma of drug use: do people use drugs, or do drugs use people? We like to say that the first is true; we act as if the second were. At the centre of the addict is the answer; perhaps for our peace of mind, it is better not to inquire too closely.

The typical young addict described in several American accounts sounds very much like the young schizophrenic, whose predicament Laing analyses so brilliantly in *The Divided Self*.[13] Both were 'good' babies, have strong but equivocal relationships with their mothers, are often apparently well looked after, but in reality were brought up as things rather than people. The schizophrenic never developed a sense of confidence in his own inner reality because no one ever 'saw' him as a valuable human being. He tries to deal with his unsureness of his own reality by constructing an unreal personality front behind which the solitary self cowers, omnipotent in a vacuum. He manipulates the false personality to fit his surroundings, in a desperate attempt to avoid the frictions and anxieties of being a rounded whole in a hostile world. (This recalls the plasticity of Chein's young addicts.) In the end the defences of his mind break down and the world invades the hollow at his centre; he becomes overtly schizophrenic. It is not impossible that opiates, by knocking out the anxiety which forces these manoeuvres, save the addict from schizophrenia and tide him over the years of internal dissociation. It is even possible that the incipient psychotic who chooses drugs is in a better position than one who tries to cope alone, for there is strong evidence (see p. 154) that heroin addiction is a phase of life from which the addict slowly matures. Although it is often, and probably quite correctly, said that drug use never improves the addict's immediate social adaptation or efficiency, this leaves out of account the slow and irretrievable personality collapse he might suffer if his drugs did not put his problems on ice until he matures from under them.

4
Attitudes to Opiates

In contemporary Western society it takes a deliberate act of the will lasting between weeks and months to become dependent on heroin. It is a definite step, taken perhaps because of a feeling of uselessness and despair, but still something well this side of suicide. The addict must have some positive hope of his involvement in drugs; to him, if to no one else, they offer some improvement on his present condition.

At some point in time, then, he was offered a shot, and accepted it. What just then was he thinking? One ex-addict, an intelligent twenty-five-year-old journalist, says: 'I was so desperate, I was in a mood to try anything. He said this would make things alright, so I took it.' In his case, the hope that heroin would help him was justified: 'The thing about H – it makes it unnecessary to worry about the things you have been worrying about. So you stop worrying, but the very fact you're not worrying means you don't have to worry. So after a bit I didn't need H, and I gave it up.' Another, an eighteen-year-old girl, who when talking about drugs affects so strong an American accent it is almost impossible to understand her, says: 'I was married at seventeen. One evening I went over to Fulham for a smoke. But there wasn't any, and I came back early. There the bastard was in bed with this bird. I felt so terrible I went back to this pusher and begged him for a shot.'

These stories tally with the American evidence on the first steps in addiction, though one should remember it is in the addict's interest to dramatize the circumstances of his beginning, and to minimize his own conscious choice. The ordinary person wouldn't think of using heroin to solve emotional problems; nor would he expect to be able to get away with a single shot. The addict, one must suppose, was potentiated towards the drug; his expectations must have differed radically from those of the rest of us. For one thing, he must have known, and have got used to, heroin as a reliever of anxiety. This argues contact with addicts and the addict culture, a contact that is anyway necessary to get illicit supplies.

For some, addiction started with the need to help themselves in an emotional crisis. What came afterwards, in the pain of the moment – so they would have us believe – was hardly considered. For others the sequel must have been more apparent. To them the drug-dependent life must have appeared attractive in itself, both from observation and from its image in our folk-lore. It is perhaps worth considering briefly the mythology of addiction; the stories people tell about it must be important influences on the decisions of new addicts.

We hardly have an indigenous junkie culture. *The Man with the Golden Arm*, *The Connection*, the beatniks are all importations. To find the name and the image of junkie, we have to go to the city bohemias of New York and Chicago where the legends are brewed.

With the Harrison Act outlawing narcotics in 1914 and a rising atmosphere of repression in America that led to Prohibition in 1920, the situation was set for the invention of the junkie as an anti-hero:

> They call him Jerry the Junker
> He's down in Chinatown
> Raggetty clothes and torn shoes
> How that boy can sing the blues
> Everything just seems to ooze
> From Jerry the Junker ...
>
> The Jury found him guilty
> And sentenced him to die ...
> They strapped him in the electric chair
> 'Twas time for him to die ...
> Ten thousand volts went right through him
> He didn't bat an eye.
> They tried a thousand times
> They heard the warden cry
> Hey, what's the use, turn off the juice
> My electric bill's too high.[1]

51

This irreverent turned into the dark, helpless, oriental dream-figure who magically soars in squalor above the capitalist world, transforming its cruelty and materialism to his spiritual advantage: Dean Moriarty, of Kerouac's *On the Road*, pirouetting in a bourgeois sitting-room:

> ... they all sat around looking at Dean with lowered and hating eyes, and he stood on the carpet in the middle of them and giggled – he just giggled. He made a little dance. His bandage was getting dirtier all the time; it began to flop and unroll. I suddenly realized that Dean, by virtue of his enormous series of sins, was becoming the Idiot, the Imbecile, the Saint of the lot.[2]

By being mad and naughty enough one escapes completely from the deadening links of the middle-class moral code and regains one's innocence. There was something in common between the beatnik and the holiness of the madman in Muslim cultures: one free of earth's chains, possessed by a being more than man-size. Moriarty is unique; for him drugs are unnecessary, but with them even the mediocre spirit can rise to his heights.

Inverted, this view of drugs is a let-out: 'Man, wouldn't I love to lead a decent life – all us junkies would. But man! Don't you see? I'm a junkie, I'm hooked, I can't get away, I can't wash/earn a living/get up/make the breakfast/pay income tax. I need my shots. Oh monkey, get off my back, man.'

This is one image of drugs – as a release. Another sees them as the mark of an esoteric world where few dare to go. One of the first 'addicts' I met was a pale eighteen-year-old from Leeds who had stupefied himself on barbiturates, but insisted he was a real junkie. He carried, to prove the point, a gigantic chromium-plated veterinary syringe for injecting high-class cows. He had never used it, nor would dare to.* Zinberg and Lewis quote the case of an American jazz musician who was admitted to hospital a second time with hepatitis. Since he used junkie slang in his speech, it was suspected that he might be an addict – always a delicate point in American medicine where ignorance might lead one to treat withdrawal as the symptoms of quite another disease, but inquiry could cause nasty scenes. This character admitted

*See p. 58, needle addiction.

shamefully that he had tried heroin twice and hadn't enjoyed it either time; he begged his doctors not to tell his wife or family since he would lose the status of being hooked. His need for psychic dependence on a drug – any drug – was so great that they could get him to abide by the regimen for hepatitis only by convincing him this too was being hooked and added to his strength and character.[3]

The same sort of effect in a suburban American environment:

Then came the first break. My good friend's mother found his paraphernalia – you know, needle, eye-dropper. She went to my father, and my father took me for a ride. He was very understanding. I finally broke down, admitted I was using drugs, said I never would again. And of course, I no sooner left him than I made a phone call to my friend – 'You better cool it' – and that night we got loaded.... So here we are, alien figures in the broad community. And somebody's mother called the police and they busted in an apartment where we were sitting, fixing, and it hit the newspapers. Because this was something new in this community. And it rocked them. Here – my God! – children in a reasonably well-to-do community using drugs. The high school was rocked. Right off the ground. The worst thing they'd had was hub-cap stealing. So – the arrest, go to jail, and of course in jail meeting a lot of people, making new connexions, friends, where to get drugs later, how to go about it, new ways of making money, and – you know, don't pretend you're naïve, pretend you're pretty slick, because that's the scene here. Then going away. To Lexington, Kentucky. Come back and my father sent me to a private school and for a few months I wasn't using drugs. Thought about it often. Thought about my old friend and wished he was around so I could show him what I knew now as a result of my nine months at Lex. I could really put him down. He wasn't hip any more ...[4]

The need of the young to be *hip* (addicts' jargon meaning to be an initiate, to have a sore on the hip from lying on boards to smoke opium; hence *hipster* skirts and trousers) probably prompts many English teenagers into experimenting with drugs. This reflects the still appalling lack of cultural opportunity in this country for teenagers, particularly from the lower classes, who in a world of experts and expertise feel doomed to stay numbered units in a mass. The need of the young for individuation and identity is acute; drugs offer them one solution. It is unfortunate that this motive is likely to be most compelling for just those inadequate, unsure, standardless personalities who seem to be particularly susceptible to drug dependence. Here are two London comprehensive school sixth-formers talking about the kids at their school who use drugs (the Greyfriars slang is their own).

It's always the real weeds, the soppy little idiots who think it's big and smart to pull out a handful of pills; and if one of them gets a shot of horse the others just die of envy, and he goes around showing off, taking his friends into the lavatory to see the needle mark on his arm. It's pathetic, I can tell you.

Drug dependence is a very complicated and multi-sided problem; there are other attractive images besides escape or glamour. One perpetual problem of adolescents is to find new forms of rebellion which will vex their elders without hurting themselves. The favourite adult image of the crazed drug fiend insolently slipping the needle into his arm, then with fearful passions, his eyes glowing like radio valves, sallying forth to wreak his filthy will on young and old alike, plays straight into the teenagers' hands. A flirtation with drugs is a marvellous way of promoting alarm among the grown-ups.

Another image of drugs, which is energetically put about as a deterrent, shows the squalor, misery and degradation of the life they cause. This too can attract, and perhaps powerfully. The potential addict, identityless, unloved, mumbles to himself: 'If it can't go right, I'll make it all go as wrong as possible'; hoping by his immolation to force others to recognize and help him. A perceptive girl who lives among addicts in Paddington says, 'I think with a lot of them it's a sort of silent cry for help'; an expression of the urge everyone has to pile on the agony until someone *has* to pick us up. Here again the American image of the junkie is the operative one, the ultimate in degeneration. Alex Trocchi describes it, from experience:

Junkies in New York are often desperate. To be a junkie is to live in a mad-house. Laws, police force, armies, mobs of indignant citizenry crying mad dog. We are perhaps the weakest minority that ever existed; forced into poverty, filth, squalor, without even the protection of a legitimate ghetto ...[5]

The self-indulgent melancholy of the adolescent is anyway one of his sharpest pleasures. The Rolling Stones sing 'This will be the last time ... I'm sorry girl, but I can't stay ... there's too much pain and too much sorrow.' To embark on heroin is, in the eyes of the world, to commit suicide; and the addict has the pleasure of being around to see the effect of finality. He hugs the catastrophic image of the junkie; there is perhaps not so much difference between him and the young Christian martyr: both by desperation invite the saving hand of the Father.

The British Addict's Life

The new addicts' manner of living seems so much a mechanism for stating their attitudes towards themselves and society that it seems more appropriate to discuss it under this heading than any other. In the Welfare State it is difficult to reach the heights of self-immolation of the classical American drug user. Heroin and cocaine are available free, in maintenance doses, from Drug Treatment Centres (see below, p. 176). By the middle of 1970, the new control system had begun to bite, and the black market price of heroin had risen to £4 to £5 from the £1 a grain it had cost over the previous five years. As a result, users switched to other drugs, particularly the more easily obtainable barbiturates which could be got in large quantities from G.P.s and ordinary hospital out-patient departments by telling a few simple lies. In law an addict under the care of a doctor is sick; if the doctor will issue the necessary certificate he can draw National Assistance and, if his card is stamped, National Insurance benefit. However, this probably seldom happens, although it would be cheaper for society to finance the addict lavishly than to let him make his own living by selling surplus drugs to converts. It is easy enough for him to make £2 a day at least in this manner. Shoplifting too is a not insuperably difficult way of supplementing one's income, and in fact many big shops have at best a neutral attitude to this offence: it does prove the attractiveness of the goods displayed. The drug-dependent personality shows a strong self-destructive streak; one feels it is almost difficult to find the situations in England for it to work on.

It has been remarked that the most striking characteristic of the new adolescent addicts is their desire for publicity. The inquirer, thinking that it is going to be difficult to meet drug users, is immediately overwhelmed by them showing off their spiritual sores like medieval beggars; willing to discuss their most intimate affairs at exhaustive, and soon tedious, length. It is clearly no use being drug dependent in London unless one is seen to be so. At midnight at Boots in Piccadilly Circus the young line up ostentatiously in the light of the neons; at John Bell & Croyden's they wait discreetly inside, slouched smellily in the over-stuffed armchairs that accommodate other customers during the day. They wait for their next day's prescriptions to be dispensed; at the stroke of midnight they are released. The night I went, a policeman recommended the group of phone boxes in Vere Street, beside the little church. There was a tousle-haired lad spreading his works out on the shelf over the directories, brilliantly lit and framed in the dark street. He slowly cooked up his dose over a stub of candle, moving to keep his back to me. Then with quite a sense of drama, he threw down his trousers and stabbed himself in the buttock with a big shiny syringe. Then he pulled up his trousers, collected his apparatus and limped briskly away. Nothing could have been more calculated for display; someone who is still injecting intra-muscularly is hardly likely to need his shot so badly he can't wait to get home.

The knowledgeable addict – in this case a writer – pursues a different system. He entertains his visitors with the ritual of the fix; boils up a pill of heroin in a medicine bottle – tension, will the glass break in the flame? Then he wraps a mysterious, spittle-wetted strip of paper round the nose of an eye-dropper, produces a hypodermic needle and shoves it over the paper. Then he sucks up the dissolved heroin into the dropper and balances it precariously on the edge of the table. Another cliff-hanging situation: will it fall? But the intrepid Scotsman coolly removes his belt – more tension, the trousers – then winds it round his left bicep. Pulling it tight with his teeth, he massages up a vein in the crook of his elbow, and then with great delicacy slides the needle into the swollen vessel. Here he explains the advantage of the dropper – the pressure of the thumb and forefinger in expelling the liquid balance each other and act across the axis of the needle, so it neither goes in nor comes out. The pressure needed to work an ordinary syringe tends to drive the needle through the vein and into the elbow joint where the heroin does little good, and invariably causes pain. That all the drug cannot be squeezed out of the eye-dropper is also turned to advantage: the belt is released and the arm allowed to fall; pulsing, the dropper fills with blood. He squeezes this back, lets it fill, squeezes and whips the needle out letting a little spurt of blood run down his arm. He dries this 'splash', conversing casually of other matters.

Many addicts here – where it is no offence to possess needles and syringes – carry a set about in an ornate spectacle case. Often they have two or three barrels and half a dozen needles, and spend as much time selecting the one to use as a golfer over his clubs. It is part of the daring never to sterilize the needles or to wash out the barrels; most of them occasionally get abcesses, blood poisoning or jaundice. But they claim to be unusually healthy – perhaps because they cannot feel the aches of ordinary mortality. In spite of this internal well-being it is easy enough, by sleeping rough and eating irregularly, wearing dirty clothes and not bothering to shave or comb one's hair, to look adequately dilapidated. 'I wear these dark glasses,' said one who came to tea with me in December 'just so people know I'm a junkie. You've got to work at the image, man.' And another, who refused to be photographed with her dark glasses on in case her parents should identify her, insisted on having a picture taken of her eyes: 'Them's real junkie's eyes, man,' she cried as she whipped off the shades.

One of the problems of dealing with drug users is that only by keeping them under observation in a ward for several days can one be sure that they are in fact dependent on drugs. Several of the 'addicts' I met seemed to be claiming the status without risking the substance, and perhaps were using the drug society as a way of escaping from middle-class living. There is a common and not unhealthy adolescent urge to get away from the paraphernalia of adult life, and to try existence at basics. The ex-addict quoted on page 50 said: 'As long as you eat and sleep, you're ahead of the game. Anything else in this life is a bonus.' Some young people get away from civilization by joining university expeditions to Samarkand; others buy a needle.

The business of getting drugs, and the very positive act of injecting them, becomes the way and the purpose of life for many users. Often it seems that the ritual is more important than the drug: one who was photographed for a magazine article ran through the routine – at his own suggestion – five times, injecting himself with tap water each time. When hard drugs became scarce during 1970, users were reported to be injecting themselves with a bizarre variety of things: crushed barbiturate capsules, aspirin, milk, and even mayonnaise. Every shot is, to the person dependent on drugs for his satisfactions, something beneficial and tangible wrung from a world that theoretically does not want him to have it. The dose gives manifold satisfaction. The person who is willing to devote his waking hours to organizing or talking about this performance, as many addicts do, is not surprisingly limited in more conventional social directions. As one moves over the spectrum of addictions, from those who are content with late hours and loud music to those who need pills, cannabis, heroin – that is, as the social machine sorts out the more disturbed – so one finds greater single-mindedness and less ability to relate to others. The couple described here, Karen and Hector, are not heroin users. In fact their chosen drug is methedrine, an amphetamine with quite the reverse pharmacological effects. But they live in the generalized drug society of Paddington and Bayswater and show its character so clearly that they are better models than many of their dopier friends.

A week after Hector had come to tea, we visited him at the room in one of the new blocks of expensive bed-sitters by the Bayswater Road, which he shared with his girlfriend Karen. They'd saved up their evening shot until we arrived, so they could do it in public. They were both chattering like children, each intent on his own story and paying no attention to the other. He says, with the air of one announcing that he'd won a prize: 'You know last week I said I was going to knock off the methedrine? Well, I've decided not to.' They get out huge anaesthetist's syringes, and Karen gets set for her injection with all the fuss of a prima donna at her toilette. She uses a fine chiffon scarf, lifted from Harrods, as a tourniquet. She is a lean blonde, about twenty-two, wearing a dress by Quant. With an ineradicable tinge of Whitechapel in her voice, she claims to be a by-blow of aristocracy. She luxuriously tickles the enormously swollen vein in her left elbow with the needle, slipping it in, then pulling it out again. After their shots they begin to talk louder and louder, pacing the tiny room like caged animals. 'What's it like?' says Hector. 'You know butterflies in your stomach? This is like having a golden eagle there.' He tries to make coffee and gets muddled; I take over and surreptitiously use hot water out of the geyser, because Karen has a reputation for spiking people's drinks with methedrine – a sleepless night is not desired. Once she stabbed a girl in the bottom while they were standing at a bar, and gave her an enormous shot.

Soon the noise became unbearable, and we left them to their happy, uncomprehending chatter.

The next evening Hector rings up in misery. Someone has stolen all their drugs, can they come over? I say, yes of course. He asks if I'll fetch them, and I say no because my wife's away with the car; he asks if I'll pay for a taxi, and I say no because she has all the money. So they come in a taxi, bound in cheerfully saying there he is, pay him. Since I can't, the taxi-driver goes away and gets a policeman. The three argue on the doorstep. In the sitting-room Karen turns out her handbag and sorts through her shoplifted heirlooms: a pair of white sea-boot socks, three presentation pen stands and sets, some battered paperbacks, including Camus' *La Peste* in French, five lighters – she wants to sell me one – a morocco spectacle case containing her works, and a green cardboard box full of empty methedrine capsules. The policeman looks in sourly, and tries to interest me in the cab driver's trouble. Then Hector gives him the address of his mother. Earlier he'd claimed that her knowing he was a junkie had broken him up.

No. 4461
85th Year 6d.

THE PEOPLE

Sunday, April 17, 1966

THE PAPER THAT LOOKS AHEAD

FRANK
FEARLESS
FREE

B.B.C. IN A WILD 'DRUG PARTY' SENSATION

ONE of the wildest parties ever held in London took place in a flat in exclusive Cheyne Walk, Chelsea, last night.

As a camera team filmed the scene on behalf of the B.B.C.'s "24 Hours" programme, some teenagers in the milling crowd puffed at doped cigarettes and others sniffed drugs from glass phials they broke.

Only a minority of the party-goers took drugs. Others just allowed themselves to run wild.

SOME DRESSED IN NOTHING AND pretended to swallow what appeared to be mothballs.

SOME POURED PAINT on sheets of paper, then put on block and sheets of paper on the polished wood floor and...

By Trevor Kempson

● Below — A "People" picture of the amazing shambles at the B.B.C. microphone is on the left.

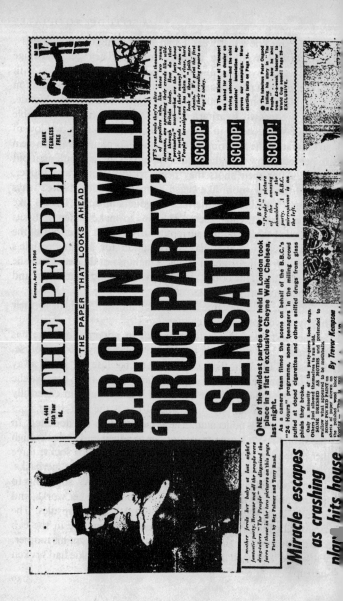

IT'S your souls they're after ... the thousands of gospellers who, like these two young Normans, are spreading their creeds like wild-fire. They disguise as "persuaders" — what are the facts about their methods ... and their money? A team of "People" investigators have written and look at three "faith merchants." We print the first of several revealing reports on Page 2 today.

SCOOP!

● The Minister of Transport has asked for our dossier on driving schools—and the chief constables' association approves our campaign. More startling facts on Page 14.

SCOOP!

● The famous Peter Osgood is back ... He is in "The People" ... Now he tells from 25-a-week labourer to £100-a-week Soccer star!—EXCLUSIVE.

SCOOP!

'Miracle' escapes as crashing plane hits house

A mother feeds her baby at last night's fantastic party. Because not all the party-goers are drug-takers "The People" has disguised the faces of those in the two pictures on this page. Pictures by Rex Palmer and Terry Rand.

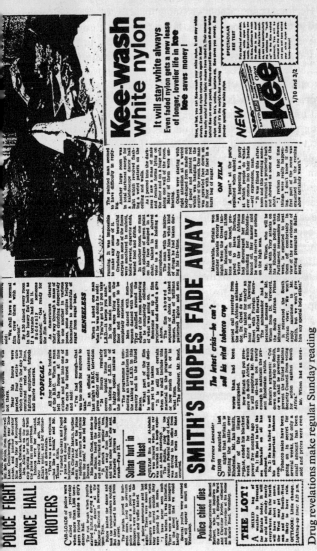

POLICE FIGHT DANCE HALL RIOTERS

CAR-LOADS of police were fighting with more than 1,000 teenagers rioted outside a city's dance hall.

The riot began when youths started fighting with the manager "pop dance" at the Market Ballroom in Berwick-on-Tyne.

Police halted the dance and the teenagers streamed out. But they refused to move from outside.

The youths, joined by hundreds, drove up to seventeen police cars and a police van. Women and children inside shops and traffic halted.

A police spokesman said last night that 1,000 teenagers were at the dance, when they were joined by a lot more.

"They were fantastic. It was fantastic. There were so many of them in so small a space, it was hardly room"

Several men were arrested and will appear in court on Wednesday.

Police chief dies

Police Superintendent Samuel Herbert, who last night was in view of his retirement, and Christine Keeler, collapsed and died yesterday at his home.

THE LOT?

A MIXED bag of weather is forecast for Britain today. It will be rainy everywhere. But the North will have sleet or snow as well as the South-West will have the mildest day. OUTLOOK: Little change.
Lighting-up time: 4.25 p.m.

Circulation clock is was there.

Near his house was parked four estate cars, which contained reels of film, lighting equipment, tripods and spotlights.

'TOPICAL'

All were given the thumbs of the B.B.C. When the men left the house at nine o'clock the cars had to be turned to me and said:

"I had enough—that was too much for anyone to see."

An official statement last night a B.B.C. television spokesman said:

"24 Hours regularly produces...

"The programme is concerned with an investigation into the taking of L.S.D. and is a highly topical nature at the moment.

"What part of the film is concerned with an editorial decision by the programme editor.

"It is still not certain whether we shall include this material in the programme or how much of it, or in what shape.

"The producer, Mr. Bond...

said:

"We shall have a normal film crew there with a director."

Sudden—
If a tornado had hit it.
Suddenly—someone packed for the film show."

SENSELESS

When I asked one man what was happening he said:

"You've got to it you take L.S.D. See what it does to it."

In the main room some couples were lying on the floor apparently to be completely senseless.

Men danced with men and women danced with women. They shuffled around the edges. One man appeared with splodges of green paint on his face, a slurred voice in a man holding a microphone.

The film showed a sequence of shots. Then patterned lights and men...

running. It was impossible to make any sense of it.

Standing by the beautiful carpets on some of the floors were munched to confetti, boiled sweets, cigarette ends, waxed food and drink.

In another room, one man with splodges of green paint on his face, talked into a chair, talked into a slurred voice to a man holding a microphone.

The man with the microphone took some of the drugs he had taken during his life-time.

The painted man seemed to have difficulty in replying.

Another large room was in a kaleidoscope dance hall light which revealed making a weird pattern on the ceiling and walls.

As I peered into the darkness I saw a mass of male and female forms lying on the floor and moved slowly along one wall of the room. There were men enmbracing.

Others were staring with rigid eyes as a nearby body-shaped form made out of paper and painted red in the centre of the room. One man was crouched down on the floor with his face in a burst bag of sugar.

ON FILM

A "guest" at the party explained when asked:

A happening is a party where nobody is a host. Whoever comes into their heads is accepted.

"It was filmed this afternoon and this evening somewhere that might happen and showed us some of the dark.

"You reckon by that time things were really happening that this is the first part of the evening we exactly wanted the evening show certainly want."

Sultan hurt in bomb blast

SULTAN Bin Ali Abdali was injured last night when he was wrecked on a bomb explosion in the Middle East.

The Sultan, said to be one of the wealthiest men, was driving to his office from his palace when the bomb exploded.

SMITH'S HOPES FADE AWAY

The latest crisis—is can't sell its vital tobacco crop

By Terence Lancaster

STONE mounted last night over the Rhodesia's prospect of winning the battle over Rhodesia. Mr. Ian Smith's regime, ended the blackest week since the break-away last December.

No. 1: The plot to beat the ban blockade on oil has failed.

No. 2: He has failed to sell his all-important tobacco crop.

Tobacco sales have been going on for less than several weeks, but only a small amount has been sold and prices were even

worse than had been pegged crop yesterday from the African section of the Wet Dr. Carel de Wet.

Now Britain will not press ahead on South Africa, which has put pressure on his regime with oil—but not nearly enough to maintain the present Rhodesian economy.

The ambassador had a harsh meeting he had faced with Tory attacks on his Rhodesian policy when he was expected to prevent the United Nations from going ahead with sanctions against Africa.

It reiterated the South African view that it will not apply sanctions to Smith, but we won't give him any special help either.

Meanwhile, Britain was making plain last night when the Greek tankers reached Mozambique, with 13,000 tons of oil which was prepared to leave Durban. Mr. Smith's officials had discouraged her from unloading her Rhodesian-bound load until he would receive new orders on the high seas.

Drug revelations make regular Sunday reading

Hector sits on the sofa groaning for a fix, rubbing his forehead and scuffing his toes on the floor. She goes through the empty phials, carried for just such an emergency, looking for a few drops of the drug. But her technique is oddly self-frustrating: she holds the little glass tubes open end down and shoves the needle up into the top – just where you would expect not to find any lurking drops. In fact she is not being constructive in the real situation, but imitating a nurse drawing an injection from a rubber-lidded drug phial, such as one might see on *Emergency-Ward 10*. 'O, Hector darling, you are so unhappy, I am so sorry for you.' She finds a couple of drops and elegantly shoots them into her own arm. She takes a dislike to me: 'Oh baby, why did we come here? He doesn't smoke, he doesn't turn on, what a drag he is. I'm so depressed – you know what I mean?' He asks for a sandwich, and she eats it. 'He treats me like a whore just because I'm a junkie and I sleep around. I've never been so humiliated in my life.' Then, in a much nicer voice, 'Can I have another sandwich please?'

Hector suggests they walk up to the West End and get some more methedrine on their new prescriptions. Then they can sell some and get a taxi back. 'Oh baby, you know I'd like to help you, you know that, but it can't be done, baby. I can't possibly walk all that way.' He suggests that he goes and comes back for her. She shoots an ugly look over her sandwich at me. 'I certainly won't be left alone with that' – Hector, defeated, starts sterilizing a sore on his arm with dabs of whisky and water. It's obvious this situation can drag on all night, so I break into the children's piggy-bank and get enough pennies for their bus fare.

Society's Attitudes to Junk

It is easy to take the addict at his word and grossly exaggerate the slavery and squalor of his life. It is an error that serves the unconscious ends of both the drug user and society.

The addict likes this image of himself because, in the main, one of his unconscious purposes in using drugs is to advertise himself in the most pitiful and hopeless light. He prefers heroin, or whichever drug he uses, to be seen as an irresistible enslavement, because this exonerates him from responsibility for his own condition. His family share the same view: 'He was a nice boy, but he got hooked,' they might say, and vow vengeance on the pusher who ensnared him – another figure necessary to the mythology. Society too prefers to think of addiction in terms of enslavement and pushers because, again, this version of the story excuses us, and makes it unnecessary to do anything very much to rehabilitate the drug user. The idea of inevitable progression from amphetamines to cannabis to opiates, though discredited by the police and the Home Office here and by authorities in America, is still another public defence mechanism which so diffuses responsibility that none have to bear it themselves. All these ideas are energetically expressed in newspaper accounts of drug use; as a journalist, I am persuaded that they reflect the feelings of a good proportion of readers.

Here, for example, is *The Times*:

PUSHERS WHO LEAD TO A SLOW SUICIDE

... Yet there remains an increasing progression from amphetamines on to heroin and cocaine, helped by smoothly operating pushers. ... 'I had been heavily on pills. They were not enough, and a fix was offered free. I took it and was hooked. The lift and feeling of detachment from a world I didn't want to face became everything. The chap who gave me the fix then charged higher and higher prices. I paid as much as £15. I registered with a doctor and my appetite increased. I would do anything, commit any crime for drugs.'

He recalled the suspicion he felt for everything and everyone, the vileness of blood spurting from a punctured vein on to a lavatory wall, the fear of being poisoned by a fumbled injection with a dirty needle.[6]

One suspects that *The Times*' reporter was, like so many who inquire from drug users, told an Irishman's tale. £15 at that time bought fifteen grains; it is unlikely that anyone could work up a habit of that size before registering with a doctor. This figure also implies spending on drugs at the rate of £5,000 a year: a rate of earning achieved only by the more successful men of business and crime, and certainly not by a doped layabout.

63

The piece goes on: 'Case histories were numerous and inevitably tragic, ending in suicide or complete physical wreckage.' This is perhaps because the untragic ones were not worth repeating, and because the drug addict's life is like a sieve: those who try heroin once and give it up, or who wean themselves from it after a few months, vanish from the scene. *They* have no reason to publicize themselves. The fit are winnowed out, and one is left with a very visible remainder of spectacularly inadequate personalities. Later the article describes the 'pathetic group of broken people' arriving at the midnight chemist to get their drugs. Even this presents a biased picture, because the sensible addict, who has not overdrawn his prescription, has no need to get tomorrow's dose at 00·01 a.m. He is asleep in his bed; only the improvident are there.

Drugs and their horrors turn up regularly as sensational features in the *News of the World* and *The People* and, regrettably, this *Times* article. Even news stories about drugs are coloured in the same way, as a few headlines show: YOUTHS BUY SEX DRUG FOR KICKS,[7] is a neat piece of sub-editor's work; and a nicely loaded suggestion comes again from *The Times*: DRUGS PREFERRED TO SEX BY YOUNG? ADOLESCENT REBELLION.[8] GIRLS STRIPPED IN SEARCH FOR DRUGS,[9] neatly links drug use with more basic and general interests.

Florid reporting, pointing out the evils of drugs in the liveliest fashion, is justified by popular commentators on the grounds that it acts as a deterrent. But it is likely that such a picture acts instead as an attraction to just the unbalanced people who are likely to become drug-dependent. Moreover, it makes it difficult for people to deal rationally with the more adjusted addict, who is prepared to work and play a more normal social part. It also confuses the distinction between drugs of quite different social potential. Everyone's interests would be better served by a more sober and rational attitude. The drug addict's presentation of himself as an infernal circus act is part of his malady; we should know better than to collaborate with him.

By 1969, perhaps because so many people's children had become actual, rather than potential junkies, boredom had set in.

Press stories about addiction to heroin were very rare, the camera teams had gone to Vietnam and then Biafra. But if less was being publicly said, far more was being done. Addiction had become a nationalized industry.

5
Sleepers

It is a curious fact that the more commonly a medical condition is found the less we know about it, and the less effort we make to find out. Ignorance of the common cold is a common jibe against doctors; on a more serious level, the effort and money devoted to the distressing but statistically insignificant thalidomide problem contrasts alarmingly with the minute funds allocated to research into schizophrenia – a malady that will affect one per cent of the population. So it is with barbiturates, the most commonly used addictive drug, with by far the most addicts. In many ways it is more pernicious than heroin, yet there is a minute literature on it, and an even smaller research effort; this is matched by only minimal public concern. For example a senior police officer at Scotland Yard, who is directly responsible for drug control in the Metropolitan area, told me that barbiturates were in no sense addictive and that they presented no problem. The Home Office considered putting barbiturates under the control of the Drugs (Prevention of Misuse) Act, 1964, when the Bill was being drafted, 'but in the absence of police or other evidence of social dangers arising from misuse, it was decided to take no action'.[1]

With this drug we have a social situation that is the reverse of those surrounding the other illicit drugs. Here abuse, addiction and suicide with the drug are taken as normal events of domestic life. Because barbiturates are prescribed by doctors to support the social system by making people tolerate ways of living that would otherwise be unbearable, society complacently accepts damage from them that would not even be contemplated from other drugs.

These dangers are nothing new.* A Dr Willcox (later Sir William Willcox) in 1913 was pointing out the perils of Veronal,

*The material in this paragraph, and much of that elsewhere in this chapter, is taken from Dr M. M. Glatt's definitive article on barbiturates in *U.N. Bulletin on Narcotics*, April–June 1962.

which had been in clinical use only ten years. Sniping went on until the fifties, when the medical press slowly awoke to the menace. An editorial in the *Lancet* saw some 'evidence that the high noon of their popularity is passing' and that the barbiturates were 'true drugs of addiction' causing a risk that was 'the least appreciated and most sinister'.[2] The *British Medical Journal* at about the same time published its own editorial warning that 'apart from the relatively slight tendency to increase the dosage compared with the behaviour of morphine addicts, barbiturates otherwise fulfil all the criteria for drugs of addiction'.[3] Even this reservation can be disputed, for patients have been seen at Lexington whose tolerance has been built up to cope with a dose of 2 gm. in twenty-four hours[4] compared with a minimum daily dose needed to establish addiction of 0·4 gm.[5]

Barbiturate-type drugs swell the outer membranes of nerve cells, squeezing the channels through which sodium and potassium ions must pass. This slows the cell's energy-producing processes, and thus the ability of the nervous system to respond to stimuli.

Barbituric acid and its homologues, the hypnotics – of which Mandrax and Trinal are the most common, with another forty different preparations in general use[6] – have effects similar to alcohol, and in general opposite to the stimulants, caffeine, amphetamine and cocaine. In terms of Eysenck's personality continuum from introversion to extraversion, a dose of the hypnotics moves a given personality towards extraversion, a stimulant towards introversion. This may sound at odds with our ordinary ideas of drug effects – a teenager who is sleepless, garrulous, phrenetic on a large dose of amphetamines may seem to be extraverted rather than introverted; but in fact the stimulants direct the attention inwards towards the thoughts and feelings of the self, rather than outwards to the environment. Thus, this book was written with the help of about four gallons of black coffee. More important perhaps than movement on the intro-extraversion scale is the effect of barbiturates on Eysenck's basic idea of inhibition. In his scheme the distinction between the introvert and the extravert is found in the quantity of 'inhibition' their nervous systems generate. Inhibition is said to be the curtain that protects the self from the world; any stimulus, any activity, generates inhibition and so automatically starts to shut itself off. Freud observed that protection from stimuli was almost more important to the organism than their reception,[7] and Aldous Huxley in *The Doors of Perception* describes the mind as a vast valve to shut off experience. In this sense, the extravert generates a lot of inhibition; he is easily bored, he needs new stimuli, and therefore appears more outgoing than the introvert who has low inhibition and is therefore satisfied longer with the same stimulus.[8] In these terms the use of barbiturates accords well with the suspicion that its abuse is largely a middle-aged, domestic affair, a characteristic of overwrought people who need to *increase* their inhibition, to free themselves from the world: people who find that life is too much for them. This may be confirmed by the popularity of barbiturates for suicide. It is significant that regular barbiturate users tend to have twice as many car accidents as the rest of us.[18] (Contrast the low accident rate of heroin users, p. 152)

Although equally serious, addiction to barbiturates differs from that to opiates in a few important respects. It seems far more destructive to personality; the barbiturate addict tends to dope himself until he is completely intoxicated – his object is oblivion. Patients who have been seen at Lexington under the influence of both opiates and hypnotics, who are said to be sensible, restrained, skilled at their jobs and to show reduced sexuality on opiates, are obstinate, aggressive, apt to masturbate in public, and full of Irish excuses for their stumbling gait and confused speech when they are on barbiturates.

Another writer describes this type of addict.

Chronic barbiturate intoxication always causes marked social and emotional deterioration. Barbiturate addicts neglect their personal appearance and are unable to work or care for themselves adequately. They are rejected by their families, lose their jobs and friends . . . They may commit crimes and not remember them. The behaviour of persons chronically intoxicated with barbiturates resembles the behaviour of chronic alcoholics and appears to be influenced to some degree by their basic personality make-up and by the mood prevailing on any given day. A barbiturate addict may be hilariously amused one day and depressed and weeping the next. Loss of emotional control frequently occurs and addicts are likely to fight over minor matters. Some individuals become infantile, weep easily, and manage to have other persons attend to their bodily needs. Others may develop paranoid ideas and in this state are somewhat dangerous. Tendencies to depression are accentuated by chronic barbiturate intoxication.[9]

The difference between this and the quietism of the heroin user is striking.

Withdrawal from barbiturates is even more catastrophic than from heroin. It can be brought on by a sudden reduction of the dose by even fifty per cent. During the first sixteen hours the patient appears to improve, becomes more coherent and behaves better. Then he becomes apprehensive and progressively weaker so that soon he can hardly stand; his hands and face begin to shake, and if his forehead is tapped above the bridge of the nose, his eyelids flutter uncontrollably. Any reflex stimulus arouses disproportionate muscular response. His temperature can rise to 105°F, his pulse rate increases by ten to twenty beats a minute. If he stands up his heart is unable to adapt and the pulse rate can rise again by up to eighty beats a minute; blood pressure falls, and these effects become more pronounced the longer he stands, so he is soon likely to faint. After this phase *grand mal* convulsions can set in. In the worst cases he screams distressingly, falls rigid to the floor, thrashes about, froths at the mouth and fouls himself. A few die at this point, but by the third day – having lost as much as twelve pounds in weight – major and minor convulsions should be over. Psychoses begin now:

Patients may see little people, giants, absent relatives, animals, insects, birds, snakes, fish and so on; and may believe that imaginary persons are trying to harm them. They may state that they have been blown up, cut with knives and forced to drink poison. The psychosis may also resemble schizophrenia . . . showing mutism, bizarre affect with ideas of control and influence, building up a system of paranoid delusions and experiencing sexual hallucinations.[9]

Usually overt signs have gone within a fortnight, although some patients have also died of exhaustion during the psychotic phase. An otherwise sane person should be more or less normal by the end of two months. As with opiates, the early stages of withdrawal can be staved off by a restoring dose.

The pharmacological danger of barbiturate addiction is increased by the character of the people who use it. Unlike heroin there is little status attached to the use of this drug, and hardly a society of addicts. No one could use opiates regularly in Britain without realizing their characteristics and identifying himself as an addict. But barbiturates are prescribed wholesale by almost every G.P. The first Brain Committee Report estimated that enough of the drug was distributed each year to provide twenty tablets a head for the entire population. So trivially is it regarded that ten per cent of this enormous output probably lies about unused in bedside-table drawers. In the Poisons Centre at Guy's Hospital there was recently a gallon glass jar filled with pills – mostly hypnotics – that had been collected from ordinary homes in ten days by a Coroner's Officer investigating sudden deaths in the north of England. Thus the barbiturate addict is able to conceal his addiction from his family, friends and even himself.* He differs profoundly from the heroin addict who uses his addiction as a characteristic defining his position in society. So it is not unusual to admit rather mad people to hospital without finding out that their condition is due to massive doses of this drug. Glatt describes a middle-aged man who was admitted in an abusive and violent state, and who developed three *grand mal* seizures in quick succession three days later. It turned out that he had been taking twelve grains of sodium amytal daily for six months to 'steady his nerves'.[15]

It has been fairly common and is now, in 1970, almost commonplace to find chronic barbiturate use in heroin addicts. About a third of all addicts admitted to Lexington, most of whom use heroin, also use barbiturates. Some are 'pan-addicts' who are so dissatisfied with their mental state that they are willing to alter it in any direction; others have become used to barbiturates because of police control of heroin. In times of scarcity, stupefaction is better than withdrawal; and in any case, in the process of

*See Evelyn Waugh, *The Ordeal of Gilbert Pinfold*, 1957.

adulterating black-market heroin, substantial doses of barbiturates are used:

> The horse [heroin] is cut with all manner of adulterous powders, until, at the average user's end, there remains 3% heroin. You can usually count on 3%. But there are times when codeine or even a barbiturate is substituted for the real thing . . . so long as they stun you, they reckon.[10]

Occasionally mystified patients at Lexington find that they are not really heroin addicts at all; their suppliers have them fooled – and hooked on an alien drug of low status.

One night I drove to meet a barbiturate addict at a crossroads in north London. I saw a gaunt man walking towards me straight across the junction of four roads. He got in the back of the car without a word, and we sat in the pale yellow sodium light. He looked terrible. People always look mauve under that light, but he looked mauver than most. His eyes went straight back in his head at the bottom of bony pits. He had a very smooth, round forehead, with a small worrying dent at the right temple. His hands galloped about in his lap, but his body sat still. He looked at me in silence, then: 'Tell me how I can get off this terrible drug.' It was easy to ask him about his addiction and the effect on his family; less easy to get sensible answers. After some minutes he said: 'Tell me how I can get off this terrible drug.'

It took a lot of questioning to discover that he had been using barbiturates illegally for four years. His epileptic brother-in-law started him off with a dose of sodium amytal. Then he had been going to an old lady doctor, getting seconal. 'It's a shame to take advantage of her really. She's eighty and she shouldn't practise because she can't even write the dates properly on the scripts. I can go in there, get eighty seconal, take a turn in the waiting room and go in and get eighty more.' He seems proud of this story and repeats it several times. He says that if he doesn't keep on taking barbiturates he gets terribly depressed first thing in the morning, and everything reels about so he can't stand up. 'I can't work, I haven't worked since February. These terrible drugs make me irresponsible.'

He has a wife and two children. A few months before a neighbour told the police that he was forging prescriptions and he was sent to hospital on probation. 'They didn't keep me long enough. Anyway, I could get out weekends and get more seconal. I even smuggled the pills back on Monday. They didn't look after us right at all.' He took me home to meet his wife, a youngish woman with a great mane of frizzy hair, and tired slitty eyes. At the moment she is calm and sensible, the room is clean, a fat four-year-old is climbing cheerfully over the furniture. The wife says: 'The police searched the place when they arrested him last time. Well, there was nothing here that shouldn't have been, but in the bedroom the Sergeant picks up this little bottle of yellow pills. "What's this?" he says, and I said, "Put them back in your pocket. I've never seen them before." When we got down the station they wanted me to make a statement, so I put in about that. They said, "Never you mind; forget that." But I wouldn't. When the statement came through typed for me to sign, there was nothing in it about the bottle.'

She says her husband hasn't been taking the drug for a fortnight now; he's finished tapering off since he came out of hospital five weeks before. He wants to find a job and a flat in another part of London where the police don't know him. He says the local ones wink at him menacingly. As I drive away I think that it is no coincidence his drug taking and his first child are both four years old. When he says, 'These terrible drugs make me irresponsible,' he perhaps means: 'I take these drugs so I can be irresponsible.'

Many cases of acute addiction – like this one – supplement their legitimate prescriptions by illegal means. But it is true to say that much barbiturate addiction is begun and encouraged by the general practitioner, of whose patients perhaps a third suffer from vague psychiatric and social troubles, inaccessible to his ordinary repertoire of remedies. Simply to stop the weeping and clear his waiting room he prescribes barbiturates. Nearly ten years ago an article in the *British Journal of Addiction* commented that there was no doubt 'barbiturates are misused on a vast scale',[11] and another, that they were used 'almost as a placebo, often to assuage the doctor's own anxieties'.[12] This is not as irresponsible as it might sound; many older practitioners were trained to regard barbiturates with complacency; and in the absence of a reliable placebo in the pharmacopoeia, they prescribe something that will have *some* psychic effect while doing less harm than many other drugs.

This can lead, however, to an unfortunate situation.

As long as the addict may be able to satisfy his demands for the drug he may feel tolerably well in spite of his symptoms, though 'persistent symptoms, particularly those accompanied by a demand for drugs'[13] might arouse suspicions. If this demand is not met the addict may suffer from symptoms such as anxiety, depression, insomnia; these temporary withdrawal symptoms may be thought to show an exacerbation of his original symptoms so that more barbiturates are prescribed, perhaps more frequently and in increasing doses. A vicious circle may set in in this manner so that an originally 'mild psychiatric disturbance is converted into a serious condition',[13] which has on rare occasions been known to lead to a leucotomy, or to several such operations. 'Patients with chronic tension states' – as Sargant writes[14] – 'may continue to remain tense and anxious for years, because they are suffering more from a self-induced or doctor-induced chronic barbiturate tension state than from a persisting anxiety neurosis *per se*. I am now seeing patients who have had one, two or even three leucotomies performed for chronic persisting tension, and who have then turned out to be, probably, cases of chronic barbiturate addiction.'[15]

These quotations are taken from articles nearly twenty years old. With the decline in the fashion for leucotomies, this unhappy fate – which, on occasion, has overtaken even chronic alcoholics, who display much the same constellation of symptoms[16] – is less likely. The younger doctor coming into general practice is probably more conscious of the dangers of barbiturate addiction, and also probably has marginally better psychiatric services to which he can refer his disturbed patients. But even so, there seems little evidence that the 'high noon' of barbiturates' popularity has passed. In 1969 barbiturates were nearly the most commonly prescribed medicine with 13·1 million scripts.[17] One bizarre result of the success of the heroin control system, started in 1968 (see below, p. 176), is that large numbers of drug users turned in

1969–70 to the easily available barbiturates. Since no injectable barbiturate preparations are available, they developed the unpleasant habit of crushing the pills, or emptying the capsules, into water and injecting the mixture directly into a vein – as with heroin. The aim, as with barbiturates taken by mouth, is to achieve stupefaction. Naturally the effects of injecting the drug are more violent, and in addition, because barbiturate preparations are very alkaline, users soon develop enormous ulcers around the site of injection.[19] It is estimated that there were, at the end of 1970, 6,000 to 8,000 people engaged in this habit.

But the place of barbiturates in public opinion is curious. Although there are 8,000 cases of barbiturate poisoning a year, although they are the second favourite means of suicide after coal gas – with ten per cent of deaths – and the favourite means of attempted suicide with nearly half of all essays, although the dangers of drinking on top of 'sleeping pills' are well known, and the dangers of addiction known anyway to doctors, barbiturates are regarded as a normal, friendly feature of life. No home is without them; and the man who crashes his car under their influence, or the woman who kills herself with a handful is reported in the papers as having 'taken an overdose'. No more need be said; we all know of what.

6
Speed

'Amphetamines, amphetamines? I do wish, Mr Er, you would not constantly confuse me with these new technical terms. Are these what we used to call "pills" in connection with juveniles?'
                                    Stipendiary Magistrate, February 1966.

The pharmacological action of this class of drug is relatively simple. By stimulating the central nervous system it produces euphoria, self-confidence, energy, alertness and endurance. There are about fifteen brands of amphetamine licitly available in England; the most common of these used illicitly, with their slang names, are: Benzedrine – *bennies*, Dexedrine – *dexy*, Methedrine – *meths*, Durophet – *black bombers*, and Steladex. Another group combines amphetamine in a mixture with barbiturate, compounding the problems of both. The principal example is Drinamyl – whose former distinctive shape gave its name, *purple hearts*; now in a new, non-heart shape, *French blue*. All of these except Durophet are manufactured by one firm, Smith Klein and French of Welwyn Garden City, which provides the bulk of the National Health Services amphetamine supplies.

Amphetamine was first prepared in 1887, and as Benzedrine, was first used medically in 1935 for the treatment of narcolepsy. The first non-medical use was in ships' survival packs during the Spanish Civil War; at about the same time it was issued to German paratroops for routine operational use. Both sides had it during the Second World War. Seventy-two million tablets were issued to British forces to be used tactically to keep troops in the line when they, and the other side too, would normally have been too exhausted to fight. Amphetamines were to be 'withheld until the men were markedly fatigued physically or mentally, in circumstances calling for a special effort'. The maximum military doses were 10 mg. in twelve hours, or 30 mg. in a week – roughly the ordinary teenager's weekend dose, but one fourth of the maximum clinical dose recommended, say, for Benzedrine.[1]

In a mild way, amphetamine is a 'superman' drug. Although the only clinical sign of having taken it is its presence in the urine, it objectively increases the capacity for simple physical and mental tasks, and increases intelligence by an average of up to eight points – as measured by simple tests.[2] However, highly co-ordinated tasks like playing golf or flying an aeroplane are unaffected in quality, though they can be prolonged beyond the normal duration.[3]

As we have seen, Eysenck finds that amphetamine moves the personality towards the introversion end of the spectrum, and decreases nervous inhibition (see p. 67).[4] As with barbiturates this finding agrees well with the characters of the people who seem to use the drug illicitly: exhausted housewives and teenagers, both groups who, as well as needing energy for their several pursuits, are also sadly bored and understimulated. They perhaps take the drug to make the most of the stimuli that are available to them. Another interesting effect, probably connected physiologically with this decrease in inhibition, is that users of the drug become more amenable to the standards and behaviour of those around them. The effect has been exploited in the treatment of disturbed and delinquent young people. Eysenck quotes a couple of American experiments, in one of which a group of disturbed children was treated with amphetamine in an institution:

During the preliminary preparations a unique opportunity for observation of each subject was afforded under conditions which required cooperation. During the period of Benzedrine medication, sociability, cooperation, attention and alertness all seemed to be improved.[5]

The drug is generally held not to be physically addictive, though for six weeks after the end of an intensive period of use some disturbance in the brain's electrical activity is reported.[6] However, this does not seem to correspond with any observable alterations to personality or mood, although the authors of the paper just referred to claim that the presence of a measurable withdrawal symptom implies genuine addictiveness. The point is, however, academic. The commonly experienced unpleasant effect of amphetamines is due simply to the way in which they increase energy. Renewed energy comes as a forced loan from the body's resources; an immediate lift lasting a few hours is followed by exhaustion and depression. If more of the drug is taken to fight off the 'come-down' the user gets himself into a bankrupt's predicament, with a large overdraft against his physical reserves. The literature on amphetamine says that exhaustion and death are likely consequences of over-use of the drug, but reported cases are so rare as to be invisible, and it seems that the majority of the minority of teenagers who use amphetamines avoid such over-indulgence.

Much is said about teenage misuse of pills; little is known. The practice seems to have started in the West End of London in 1960 or so, and became noticeable by 1963. It has spread to the centres and suburbs of most cities in the British Isles, and is, with imports from the continent guaranteeing the black market, now an apparently ineradicable part of adolescent life. The point of using the drug is to extend and intensify the weekend, a short period of escape from tedious school or dull jobs. The kids sit in beat clubs, coffee bars; they dance, talk, wander the streets, which for once they have to themselves, from Friday night to Sunday. It is probable that this intensive period of group sociability and exploration, which for a few is emphasized by amphetamines, lasts roughly two years between leaving school at sixteen and starting serious courting at eighteen.

The meagreness of the literature on this subject is shown by the continued references in scientific papers to Anne Sharpley's celebrated pieces on pill-taking in Soho published in the *Evening Standard* in the spring of 1964. Although her articles are remembered more for the exotic and desperate characters she discovered, many of her observations are moderate and intelligent.

They [the teenagers] are looking for, and getting, stimulation, not intoxication. They want greater awareness, not escape. And the confidence and articulacy that the drugs of the amphetamine group give them is quite different from the drunken rowdyness of previous generations on a night out.[7]

The important difference between purple hearts and alcohol is that

77

for the first time people in the mass are experiencing a cerebral sensation. Not a physical one. Purple hearts taken in the quantity that most teenagers take them – half a dozen to a dozen,* to keep them going over the weekend and save them the expense of hotel rooms and food – are not specially harmful. Indeed they have an enhancing effect in giving them confidence and clarity.[8]

She might have added that young girls, staying up all night, keeping awake and alert on amphetamines, with their sex drives reduced, are less likely to be seduced and made pregnant than they would be using alcohol. Since pills came into use, there has been a noticeable decline in teenage drunkenness, though one can only guess at the causal connection.[9]

One might even compare the experience and excitements of a two-day, three-night, Soho pills weekend with the central experience of an Outward Bound Course, designed for people of the same age-group. One of the high points of this character-building course is a four-day mountain expedition. Both this and the weekend make considerable demands on the individual's initiative and stamina, both expose him to dangers he would otherwise not know about, both test his self-reliance and increase his self-confidence, both by transcending his normal endurance and capabilities enlarge his knowledge of himself and the world he lives in. Accidents happen in both situations, but for the large majority no lasting harm results; the weekend on pills has the advantage that it is voluntarily chosen and relevant to urban living.

(The parallel is even closer. The psychic malleability produced by amphetamines is induced in the Outward Bound situation by exhaustion, fear, isolation and feelings of guilt due to unavoidable breaches of the Course regulations. The resulting plasticity is acted on by strong motivating pressure from the Course instructors. In effect the Outward Bound Course is a form of brainwashing consciously or unconsciously designed to bring teenage values into line with the Establishment's. The methods

*The clinical dose advised by the manufacturer for Drinamyl is three pills a day, the last not after 4 p.m. A dozen in three days hardly exceeds this; allowing that teenagers do not want to sleep, it is a dose unlikely to carry any risk of psychosis.

adopted tally very closely with Dr William Sargant's account of the best brainwashing procedures used in Russia and China; methods which he describes as being superior to the use of drugs.)[10]

The connection between amphetamines and juvenile delinquency is also somewhat exaggerated. An often quoted survey of young people admitted to a remand home showed that 18 per cent had the drug in their urine, but otherwise there was nothing to distinguish these from the 82 per cent who had not.[11] It is possible that in a few individuals the drug releases latent anti-social action, but in as many others, normally repressed and frustrated, it enables better adjustment and acceptable social behaviour. Howard, in an article whose tenor is that far more teenagers claim to have used pills than have actually done so, reports a few cases of repressed sexual deviance made actual under the stimulus of amphetamines, particularly the quick-acting methedrine – which is now unobtainable.[12] But any form of social activity throws up a few people whose behaviour is unacceptable. The police object to juvenile amphetamine use because it is thought to cause fights, because cars parked near beat clubs get scratched and children stay up all night.[13] These are all things likely to happen anyway when teenagers are allowed out all night; there is no evidence of any increase attributable solely to pills. It seems likely that the campaign against amphetamines, resulting in the Drugs (Prevention of Misuse) Act, 1964, is an attempt by adult society to seize on something concrete in the apparent morass of changing adolescent standards.

A more promising line of criminal inquiry might be into the fraud of those who supply teenagers with amphetamines. In the thriving black market the supply of amphetamines stolen off the production lines of the firms that make them, and imported – often from Spain – is supplemented by a variety of home-made and sometimes noxious substances. This aspect of the trade shows interesting analogies with the American black market in heroin. Howard[13] says that harmless powder compressed into pills is often sold as Benzedrine for 12½p a tablet; another ruse is to dye aspirins with purple ink (not easy – the surface of the pill flakes off) and sell them as a new brand of Drinamyl. Stimulants, or some colourable simulacra, are available in clubs, dance halls, coffee bars, either passed from hand to hand, or dissolved in bottles of squash. Such manoeuvres must decrease even more the customers' check on their purchases. Their distribution appears to involve a fairly sophisticated network and a hierarchy of suppliers who handle quantities of pills numbered in millions.

Apart from exhaustion, and the legal penalties attendant on possession of the drug, the chief danger of indiscriminately used amphetamines lies in habituation and psychosis. These are often, but not always, found together. A large enough dose – 50 mg. or 10 Benzedrine tablets – is said to be very likely to precipitate a psychosis lasting up to a week in any normal person.[15] (Incidentally, this seems to dispose of some teenagers' widely reported boasts that they take 100 pills at a time – exaggeration on a level with the nightly 'dozen pints' of some habitual drinkers.) Here again we touch on the mysterious connection between drugs and madness: amphetamine is thought to act in the body by competing for amine oxidase and so potentiating the body to adrenaline – an essential chemical in the brain, very similar in structure to mescaline. Also, in view of heroin's possible efficacy in preventing schizophrenia (see p. 156), it is interesting that amphetamine and the opiates cancel each other out.[3]

The symptoms of madness induced by prolonged overdoses of amphetamines are 'primarily of a paranoid psychosis with ideas of reference, delusions of persecution, auditory and visual hallucinations in a setting of clear consciousness, possibly indistinguishable from acute or chronic schizophrenia'.[14] The condition is treated by withdrawal of the drug and giving barbiturates; there is a high relapse rate, and in the physical and mental depression after large doses suicide is common. But it seems that taking doses of this magnitude is in itself a symptom of acute mental disturbance. Of forty-six cases reviewed by Connell who had been admitted to London hospitals with psychotic symptoms, 66 per cent had been treated before for psychiatric illness, 26 came from families with a history of alcoholism and psychiatric illness, and in the group that had used amphetamines for some time, everyone had used some other drug or excessive alcohol.

Some cases:

Case 6: He felt depressed and bought an amphetamine inhaler, ingesting the contents over six hours. Soon people began to look at him in a peculiar way. He began walking the streets and slept in the park. The next day he spent looking for gold in the park; stones there seemed to be gold. That evening he heard people talking about him and was sure that people were going to kill him. Cars and people followed him, and there were numerous special signs. Finally he climbed onto the roof of a building and began throwing tiles at the gang in the street below.

Case 23: There was a five-day history of wandering on a special mission for God. This was partly to test her and there were numerous special signs, special meanings and persecutory figures in this experience. She had been taking dexedrine for weight reduction and fatigue. She finally went to a relative's house in a filthy state and defecated on the carpet.

Case 29: This patient habitually ingested the contents of methedrine inhalers for depression. He began to feel that everyone was against him and heard 'pro' and 'anti' voices. Finally he felt that his wife was against him and when she threatened to leave him he became acutely depressed and sought admission to hospital.

Connell reports that a much smaller dose than is needed to produce psychosis in normal people will markedly increase the hallucinations of schizophrenics.[14] It seems likely that in some persons whose body chemistry is nearly that of the schizophrenic (often betrayed by their previous abnormal behaviour), a relatively small dose of amphetamine will tip them temporarily over the edge into a psychotic state that lasts until their precarious chemical balance is restored. The doses one could get from amphetamine inhalers before the drug was put on the Poisons Schedule 4 in 1955 could amount to a hundred times the clinical dose. Dramatic results were to be expected.

In another paper Connell reviews nine adolescents who had been referred to the Maudsley Hospital with amphetamine troubles. All had had short-lived paranoid experiences, and 'all, without exception, had problems of adolescent adjustment, and the majority had shown the beginnings of difficult behaviour before taking drugs.'[15]

Of 263 ex-Borstal boys under the supervision of the Central After-care Association in 1962, a third used or had used amphetamines, and a tenth had to 'excess'. These must represent a very small proportion of the teenage population at risk. Interestingly, the Director says that of twenty-five boys recently brought to his notice as drug users only one had had a normal home. Seven were illegitimate and in the history of fifteen of the others there was gross parental rejection.[16]

An Australian study of thirteen people dependent on the drug – who also displayed an extraordinary variety of sexual deviations – confirms the importance of original personality disturbance in forming this condition. Among these there were six cases with a family history of addiction to alcohol or drugs, and overt mental illness in seven families. Of the thirteen only four had no history of either of these, all but one had been openly rejected by their parents, and the exception had been an orphan brought up on an island by a cruel step-father. However, perhaps as nature's compensation, one couple claimed that they could, with amphetamines, prolong sexual intercourse to ten hours or more. In most people, though, the authors conclude, the drug can increase sexual desire if it is already present, but reduces performance. All these patients said they used amphetamine because it made them feel powerful, great, 'in control'.

The occurrence of marked regression and the use of passive-receptive forms of mastery indicate the presence of considerable personality defect.[17]

Another series of fourteen patients dependent on the drug showed that eleven had used other drugs to excess: morphine, bromide, barbiturate, alcohol and even caffeine. '. . . The basic reason for addiction must lie in the personality of the addict.'[18]

The published accounts of amphetamine habituation and psychosis overwhelmingly suggest that these states are, like all other drug dependence, symptoms of severe personality disorders rather than disease-like conditions that are 'caught' through bad company and the want of proper control of drugs. Hector and Karen (p. 58) are hardly normal. Tony Parker in

Five Women gives a vivid portrait of one such personality. Carol Dean, known in Soho as Carol the Pill because she would buy any quantity at any time, was a runaway from a family in a remote Cornish village. Emotionally very unstable, the only steady mark in her world was her elder sister who had earlier run away to London. Carol lived with a boy, but without sex. This is her first introduction to the pills scene:

I stayed up all night in the club, taking these pills every hour or so, and I'd never enjoyed myself so much in all my life, I felt on top of the world, as though I could go on dancing and talking and laughing for ever and ever, just listening to records on the juke box and drinking coffee.

But next morning when the pills had all gone and the effect had worn off – it was like I wanted to fall down dead, honest – you know, all the stuffing gone out of your body, your mouth dry, your head spinning, your head going a mile a minute, oh you feel shocking, terrible, I can't describe it. All I wanted was to go to bed and sleep and sleep and sleep. . . . Like I said, you don't care, when you're on the pills, what you look like or what you do, and you can get very abusive too. I was effin' and blindin' at the law when I went out of the station, for taking me in, but somehow I knew it wasn't going to be long now before they'd really got something to hang on me.[19]

Here seems to be an extremely insufficient, bleak, unstable personality who suddenly equates the use of amphetamines with the delights of the city and her own enjoyment of independence and new easy social relationships. Naturally she becomes attached to them.

The most worrying aspect of teenagers' amphetamine use is their indifference to dosage. The faith the young have, in common with their elders, that anything pharmaceutical is both safe and beneficial, is touching but ill-advised in these days of potent drugs. The regular pill-user doubtless learns his safe dose or goes under; in the process he may fall out with his family, lose jobs, get into trouble with the police. But among the recommendations of the Report of the Advisory Committee on Drug Dependence* was

* *The Amphetamines and Lysergic Acid Diethylamide (LSD)*, Report by the Advisory Committee on Drug Dependence, H.M.S.O., 1970.

this: 'The occasional oral use of a pep pill ought to be regarded as much less serious than the injection of amphetamine which is as dangerous as any form of drug abuse.' Injection of a liquid preparation, methedrine, became a problem in 1967, and when, from April 1968, heroin could only be got from clinics, the methedrine 'misuse problem soon reached epidemic proportions'. Methedrine was quickly taken off the market (see below, p. 178). Of all the drugs which are abused in Britain, methedrine was probably the most troublesome. Users would be violent, insulting, criminal under its influence (see above, p. 80). Several hospitals and social work schemes dealing with drug users have reported that their lives became much easier after it was banned.

More serious perhaps than adolescent extremism, is domestic habituation to amphetamines. Prescription of these drugs is not on the vast scale as for barbiturates, but still amounts – with 3·75 million scripts in 1964 – to 1·79 per cent of all prescribing.[20] This is in spite of a general decline in their use in hospitals, and a medical disenchantment with their efficacy. Oswald and Thacore wrote eleven years ago: 'Therapeutic indications for amphetamine are today becoming vanishingly small'[6]: diet is best for obesity, they are no use in endogenous depressions and there are better things for narcolepsy. But again, like barbiturates, they are used by G.P.s and psychiatric out-patient departments almost as placebos, simply to do something for the vague miseries that abound in our society. A survey of the prescriptions for the forty or so preparations that contain amphetamines was made in Newcastle-on-Tyne for May and November 1960. About 200,000 tablets were prescribed each month on some 4,000 scripts. Expressed as a proportion of all prescriptions in these periods for this area, these come to 3·4 per cent. A detailed inquiry showed that no more than one per cent of registered patients were being prescribed amphetamines regularly; so that roughly 2,600 people were being given 77 tablets each a month. It was estimated that 20 per cent of these, or 520, were in fact dependent on the drug, had used it a long time, and strongly resisted its withdrawal.[21]

It is interesting to try to estimate from this work how many people there might be in England and Wales who are dependent on amphetamines. There are formidable statistical difficulties and at the best we can only come within an order of magnitude. The Newcastle prescribing rate for amphetamines, at 3·4 per cent, is considerably higher than the national rate for amphetamines. But we can perhaps correct this by making the otherwise arbitrary assumption that amphetamine misuse is a feature of urban life. About half the population of England and Wales lives in towns of more than 100,000 inhabitants.[22] In Newcastle we had a year's total of 2,400,000 prescriptions associated with 520 people dependent on amphetamines. Applying this relationship to half the year's prescriptions for the whole country – 104·7 million scripts – we get a figure of 23,000 people who are likely to be dependent. It is unfortunate that Drinamyl is so popular – 53 per cent of the prescriptions in Newcastle were for it – because it is an amphetamine–barbiturate mixture; the psychic dependence that can be formed for any drug can be complicated here by genuine physical addiction to the barbiturate component.

In Newcastle, 85 per cent of those who had the drug regularly were women, housewives like this unfortunate:

> I started taking the tablets about three and a half years ago when I felt I could not get through my housework after working in the mill. At first I only took half a tablet a day. They made me feel fine and I was much better tempered with the children. But gradually I needed more and more – I could not get enough from my own doctor and used to wait until he was away and then go to other doctors who were acting for him. Plenty of housewives are taking these tablets. It is the only way they can get through, especially if they have to go out to work.[23]

She was twenty-eight with five children, had been put on probation for fraudulently getting prescriptions for Drinamyl, and was sent to hospital for a year to be 'cured'. Her children were put in the care of the local authority. Who should be blamed: the drug, a weak personality, our society where the mother of five small children has to go to work?

Another woman, looking after her husband and five children

in a minute flat, was charged with forging a prescription to get 136 Drinamyls. She is forty-seven and said,

> They seemed to do me a lot of good. Without them I don't seem to have the energy to cope with things. There is a lot more work to be done since the baby arrived six months ago. At normal times I need about three a day, then I can face problems in the house much better.[24]

An interesting and well-constructed recent inquiry in Liverpool into domestic Drinamyl dependence found that although 58 per cent of a sample of patients who were regularly being prescribed these pills said 'they could not do without them', more than half of these, or 30 per cent of the whole sample, were just as satisfied with blue heart-shaped dummy tablets. Of the rest, who said they *could* do without, a smaller proportion were deceived by the dummies. Altogether, it seems that about half the people who are regularly prescribed these tablets are likely to be just as happy with a placebo. For them the significance of the medicine probably lies in its symbolism of society's concern. Wilson and Beacon conclude:

> If general practitioners cannot obtain adequate psychiatric help for their patients, the prescription of Drinamyl to these under carefully controlled conditions cannot wholly be condemned even though the patients get habituated to it. In the case of the psychologically dependent patients, it is the act of taking the medication rather than its pharmacodynamic action which was more important, and continued prescription of Drinamyl to these patients cannot be too strongly condemned.[25]

In recent years a 'new' stimulant drug has appeared on the illicit British market: cocaine. Derived from the leaves of the South American coca plant, it has been used for centuries by the natives of the Andes to inure themselves against cold and exhaustion. It became an important part of the Spanish colonial economy when they took these mountain people down into the steamy coastal jungles to cultivate their haciendas. Without the drug the natives were useless; with it they could labour three months before they died of exhaustion and pneumonia.

A vast range of cocaine preparations were sold in America

in the latter decades of the last century: as linctus, chewing gum, syrup, nose sprays. The best-known survivor is Coca-Cola, first sold as a syrup in 1886 and advertised as the 'intellectual beverage'. The drink's characteristic flavour was produced by coca leaves, which brought with them a hefty and commercially advantageous charge of the drug, producing in the customers a psychological habituation. In 1915 cocaine was removed to prevent Southern blacks enraging themselves on it, and this state of affairs continues to this day, though the previous obligation to demonstrate the lack of cocaine to the Federal Government was removed in 1965.

The effects of cocaine are very like amphetamine: to give physical and mental energy, exhilaration, and to increase alertness and capacity for work and pleasure. Much lauded as a sex aid, it is said to increase the intensity of orgasm, while, since it is also an anaesthetic, delaying it. The sort of people who might use it are public performers – musicians, comedians, salesmen – because it gives the taker an aliveness that may be hard to procure by ordinary means. But, as with amphetamine, today's increased energy must be paid back in tomorrow's exhaustion.

It also makes prolonged exertion possible and was much favoured by nineteenth-century armies to enable soldiers to withstand the fatigues of campaigning. The French Army swore by *vin Mariani*.

Cocaine has now, owing to its high price, a sort of champagne status among illicit drugs. It was last widely used in Britain on its own during the twenties.* For a fictional account of this period see Dorothy Sayers' *Murder Must Advertise*. Heroin addicts have used it for many years to remove the dulling effect of the opiate.

The U.S. Commission on Marihuana and Drug Abuse found in 1973 that 10 per cent of high-school students had tried cocaine.

*See, generally, Ashley, R., *Cocaine, Its History, Uses and Effects*, St Martin's Press, New York, 1975.

7
The Weed

Cannabis, marihuana, hashish, pot, charge, tea, ganga, grass, and ten dozen other names; the weed is now probably the most widespread illicit drug in the United Kingdom, with between 30,000 and 300,000 users.[30]

The marihuana plant is a relative of European hemp, looks rather like a scrawny, six-foot nettle, and grows well anywhere hot. Although it is cultivated under glass in several parts of England, notably round Windsor, the best supplies come from the Middle East, North and West Africa, India and the West Indies. The dried leaves – tea or pot – are smoked as or with tobacco in cigarettes or pipe-like devices; the resin distilled from the sticky flowers is made up into cakes that look rather like Oxo, are called hashish, and are used crumbled into cigarettes.

Its effects are well known. As seen from the outside it produces a very characteristic reddening of the eyes, dryness of the mouth, increase in appetite, and the subject 'exudes a strong odour of burning grass'. The physical signs are slight and unimportant, compared to the spectrum of mental effects:

... (a) dulling of attention, (b) loquacious euphoria of variable duration, (c) usually some psycho-motor activity and affective lability coloured by the underlying personality [i.e. emotional reactions are likely to become misplaced or misdirected – an example with another drug, alcohol, would be flirtations at a cocktail party], (d) perhaps some distortion of perception and time sense, depending on the dose, (e) perhaps some lassitude culminating in deep sleep if the dose is sufficient.[1]

Although cannabis is more closely related to the hallucinogens than to any other drug, Michaux, after repeated experiences with both, writes: 'Compared to other hallucinogenic drugs hashish is feeble, without great range, but easy to handle, convenient, repeatable without immediate danger.'[2] Théophile Gautier gives a classic account from the inside:

My body seemed to dissolve and I became transparent. Within my breast I perceived the hashish I had eaten in the form of an emerald scintillating with a million points of fire. My eyelashes elongated indefinitely, unrolling themselves like threads of gold on ivory spindles which spun of their own accord with dazzling rapidity. Around me poured streams of gems of every colour, in ever-changing patterns like the play within a kaleidoscope. My comrades appeared to me to be disfigured, part men, part plants, wearing the pensive air of Ibises. So strange did they seem that I writhed with laughter in my corner and, overcome by the absurdity of the spectacle, flung my cushions in the air, making them twist and turn with the rapidity of an Indian juggler.

The first attack passed and I found myself in my normal state without any of the unpleasant symptoms that follow intoxication with wine. Half an hour later I fell once more again under the domination of hashish. This time my visions were more complex and more extraordinary. In the diffusely luminous air, perpetually swarming myriad butterflies rustled their wings like fans. Gigantic flowers with calyxes of crystal, enormous hollyhocks, lilies of gold or silver rose before my eyes and spread themselves about me, with a sound resembling that of a firework display. My hearing became prodigiously acute. I actually listened to the sound of the colours. From their blues, greens and yellows there reached me sound waves of perfect distinctness. A glass inverted, the creak of an armchair, a word pronounced in a deep voice, vibrated and rumbled about me like the vibrations of thunder. My own voice seemed so loud that I dared not speak for fear of shattering the walls with its bomb-like explosion. More than five hundred clocks seemed to announce the hour in voices silvery, brassy or flutelike. Each object touched gave off a note like that of a harmonica or an aeolian harp. Floating in a sonorous ocean, like luminous islands, were motifs from *Lucia* and the *Barber of Seville*. Never has greater beauty immersed me in its flood. . . .[3]

And so on; a vision of a world so fantastic and charming that one is averse to follow him there, for fear of trampling on his silver flowers. It is interesting that he describes synaesthesia – 'the sound of the colours' – the crossing of perception from one sense to another, which is very characteristic of the LSD-

induced state. Baudelaire, another member of the Club des
Haschischiens which used to meet at the Hotel Pimodan in the
Latin Quarter of Paris in the mid nineteenth century, emphasizes
that the hashish hallucination transforms the real world rather
than – as we find with LSD – creating an unreal internal world.
The hallucination is progressive, almost voluntary, and ripens
only through the action of the imagination. Sounds may seem to
say strange things, but there always was a stimulus there in the
first place. Strange shapes may be seen, but before becoming
strange the shapes were natural.[4]

The drug's exotic and euphoric effects accorded perfectly with
the floridity of Parisian intellectual life a century ago. The wonders of the East were being unfolded, the French were colonizing
Africa and fertilizing themselves with Arab culture. Doctor
Moreau de Tours brought *dawamesc* from Algeria – a mash
made up of hemp plant tops, sugar, orange juice, cinnamon
(itself a marihuana-like drug), cloves, cardamom, nutmeg, musk,
pistachios and pine kernels – and, balancing on the little green,
smelly nuggets, the Club made strange voyages. It is likely the
common dose then was far larger than smokers get today. Lud-
low, the young American who published the anonymous *Hasheesh
Eater* in 1860, reports that he took fifty grains at a time, a quantity which would now be called a severe overdose, and that the
effects lasted for days. A medical volunteer in a recent experiment
took forty-eight grains, grievously twitted his superior on his
newly acquired Fellowship of the Royal College of Physicians,
and felt for a while that 'time and space seemed compressed into
one bright minute, during which all was gay talk, and myself the
carefree centre of it all.' Dosed with largactil and intravenous
dextrose – the insertion of the needle was exquisitely painful – he
recovered within three days. The fatal dose is said to be about
one and a half pounds of hashish.[5]

An experienced smoker, who stops when he has reached the
peak of euphoria, is unlikely to feel the effects of the drug for
more than eight or ten hours, will hardly experience the excitement of the Club, and will suffer no hangover. His experiences

while the effect lasts are very much dependent on his mood to begin with, because, like alcohol, marihuana intensifies one's original state of mind. William Burroughs says: 'depression turns to despair, anxiety to panic, it makes a bad situation worse.' It is impossible therefore to say that cannabis either does or does not produce crime, sexuality or indeed any particular social effect. These forms of behaviour are at several unpredictable removes from the centres of action of the drug in the brain; character, training, social situation, all are involved in the drug user's final behaviour as society sees it.

Intellectually, the drug increases imagination but reduces concentration.[6] Intelligence-test scores are slightly lower or unchanged, and if attention is held, say in a game of poker, an expert player can more than hold his own against other good players.[7] Jazz musicians claim that they play more excitingly under the influence than without; in simple – but musically sterile – laboratory tests of note identification and beat duration their performance is worse on the drug.[6] A group of painters and musicians, asked to map out a programme of activity before taking the drug, and then left to themselves under its influence, failed to achieve anything.

It is worth quoting this rather moving letter from a woman to the Canadian Commission of Enquiry into the Non-Medical Use of Drugs, and printed by them in their interim report:[31]

In his bid to solve the 'generation-gap' our middle son brought a packet of marihuana to us for a Christmas present a year ago. I was slightly horrified because I hoped, like most other parents, that my children were not using it. I was not prepared to try it then. However, with the same sort of persuasion that had previously won him the permission to keep a live garter snake, paint his room in odd colours, and study art instead of mathematics, I tried it as did his father, brother and sister.

Not too much happened the first time, except that a kind of mellowness settled over the family. We smiled a lot and listened to music that seemed somehow less forbidding than when the kids played the records previously. The next night we smoked the rest of it, and the place started swinging. It was really marvellous. Everyone managed to talk together, about trivialities mainly, there was no tendency to put down anyone. Opportunities to complain or dig at the lack of academic diligence that was always part of the previous conversations with this boy were ignored, and father in particular listened to some of his ideas with a semblance of civility. That alone made the experience worthwhile. The family that night was closer together than anytime I can recall. I was greatly surprised to see that what had seemed to be many hours was only an hour and a half. We were all very happy together, and went off to our rooms feeling as if we loved each other for the human beings we were, not for mere points on a scale of achievement.

For the first time in years my husband and I talked for an hour or more about work, plans, memories, problems and possible solutions – all things we never discussed with each other because of the old scientist/ humanist conflict and the rivalries that develop between people in conflicting fields of interest. The miracle is that he seemed also to be a human being, and not only a work machine that ignored people, and particularly his family. I must have seemed somewhat more reasonable to him too, as he did not try to depreciate my interests.

The real miracle followed when we had intercourse. Instead of the dull, perfunctory act it had become, usually indulged in on my part because it made it possible to get out of it the next night, sex was something splendid. All the old routine thrust and counter thrust to get it over with as soon as possible disappeared. The sensation was extraordinary, each second was a kind of new adventure, each movement an experience, and the climaxes beautiful beyond description. It was far more beautiful than the first weeks of marriage, and the glow of fulfilment lasted throughout the next day. It was both a physical and intellectual rediscovery between two people who knew each other too well for too long.

In an important examination of the addictive qualities of cannabis a group of American prisoners were allowed as much as they wanted of a synthetic version of the drug – pyrahexyl compound – for a month. The ordinary effects were seen at first, then euphoria gave way to lassitude after a few days; the subjects became careless, their pulse and temperatures fell, and their weight increased. They found comprehension, analytical thinking and tests of manual dexterity difficult. Their inhibitions were decreased, and they were more suggestible. The dominant frequencies in their E E G traces were slowed down. On withdrawal of the drug one subject had a slight panic reaction and another a mild manic excitement, but there were no withdrawal symptoms and no demands to continue.[6]

Recently there has been some interest in Eastern Europe in cannabis as an antibiotic. It is reported to be active against gram-positive organisms at one part per 100,000. But since it is ineffective in the bloodstream, it seems that its use is confined to ear, nose and throat conditions.[8]

Marihuana as a Social Menace

The social position of no other drug is as equivocal as that of cannabis. It is variously represented as a vicious scourge or a harmless diversion. In both America and Britain it is controlled as rigidly as heroin, yet the *Lancet* recently ran an editorial suggesting that the indictment of cannabis was hardly proven, and that although one should be cautious in relaxing controls, the State might do better out of taxing the legalized sales of the drug than it does from fining detected illicit use.[9] Responsible doctors are prepared to publish statements like this:

I would be far happier if my own teenager children would, *without breaking the law*, smoke marijuana when they wished, rather than start on the road of so many of their elders to nicotine and ethyl alcohol addiction.[10]

Although it is very like LSD in its effects, there is little intellectual interest in it at the moment, and its use is found among relatively isolated groups.

As a matter of form, marihuana was outlawed here in 1928 when Great Britain ratified the Geneva Convention of 1925 controlling the manufacture, sale and movement of dangerous drugs – principally opiates, cocaine and cannabis. We had then no sort of social problem with the drug in this country, and no prospect of one; the ratification was simply so that we could suppress drug traffic in colonies and dependent countries. The drug first became a problem for the West in America during the hysterical thirties. Three titles from a bibliography of the period show which way the wind was blowing at all levels of sophistication:

Marihuana as a Developer of Criminals,[11] *Sex Crazing Drug Menace,*[12] *Exposing the Marihuana Drug Evil in Swing Bands.*[13]

The opposition demonstrated their intellectual degeneration in songs like this:

Sweet Marihuana Brown

In her Victory Garden
The tea grows all around,
She plants, you dig,
She flips your wig.
Get help, take care,
Look out, beware
Of Sweet Marihuana Brown.
Boy that gal means trouble
You ought to put her down
Every time you take her out
She's bound to take you in
Sweet Marihuana Brown.[14]

The marihuana scare seems to have begun in this country in the mid fifties with the emergence of the coloured immigrant as a social problem. One serious-minded work, *Indian Hemp, a Social Menace*, was published by a barrister in 1952;[15] he quotes as a crushing indictment of the drug and its users a series of articles from the *Sunday Graphic* – a now extinct journal. They begin:

After several weeks I have just completed exhaustive inquiries into the most insidious vice Scotland Yard has ever been called on to tackle – dope peddling.

Detectives on this assignment are agreed that never have they had experience of a crime so vicious, so ruthless and unpitying and so well organized. Hemp, marihuana and hashish represent a thoroughly unsavoury trade.

One of the detectives told me: 'We are dealing with the most evil men who have ever taken to the vice business.' The victims are teenage British girls, and to a lesser extent, teenage youths. . . .

The racketeers are 90 per cent coloured men from the West Indies and west coast of Africa. How serious the situation is, how great the danger to our social structure, may be gathered from the fact that despite increasing police attention, despite several raids, there are more than a dozen clubs in London's West End at which drugs are peddled.

As the result of my inquiries, I share the fear of detectives now on the job that there is the greatest danger of the reefer craze becoming the greatest social menace this country has known.

The other day I sat in a tawdry West End club. I was introduced by a member, a useful contact both to me and the police.

Drinks sold were nothing stronger than lukewarm black coffee, 'near beer' or orangeade.

I watched the dancing. My contact and I were two of six white men. I counted twenty-eight coloured men and some thirty white girls. None of the girls looked more than twenty-five. In a corner five coloured musicians with brows perspiring played bebop music with extraordinary fervour. Girls and coloured partners danced with an abandon – a savagery almost – which was both fascinating and embarrassing. From a doorway came a coloured man, flinging away the end of a strange cigarette.

He danced peculiar convulsions on his own, then bounced to a table and held out shimmering arms to a girl. My contact indicated photographs on the walls. They were of girls in the flimsiest drapings.

'They are, or were, members,' I was told.

We went outside. I had seen enough of my first bebop club, its coloured peddlers, its half crazed, uncaring young girls.

In their way, the pieces are small masterpieces of mass Sunday indignation; but one feels they come to the *point d'appui* only at the end of the last article:

'The day will come,' said the dusky Jesse, 'when this country will be all mixtures if we don't watch out. There will be only half castes.'[16]

The book goes on to suggest with legalistic subtlety that cannabis could be the instrument of the perfect crime – a secret dose, a psychosis, committal to mental hospital, a power of attorney – Heavens, the deed box! Exactly the fantasy that is advanced against L S D now.

Investigations into the Social Effects of Cannabis

The first properly conducted inquiries into the effects and harm done by the drug seem to have been those of the U.S. Army in the Canal Zone in 1932–3.[17] It was concluded that marihuana presented no threat to military discipline, and 'there is no evidence that marihuana as grown here is a habit-forming drug in the sense in which the term is applied to alcohol, opium, cocaine, etc. and that no recommendations to prevent the sale or use of marihuana are deemed advisable.'

Indeed Murphy, reviewing the recent psychiatric literature in the W.H.O.'s authoritative *Bulletin on Narcotics*, says:

The majority of the papers here reviewed hold fairly clearly that cannabis is 'habit forming' rather than 'addiction producing' (in terms of the now obsolete W.H.O. definitions). Most individual users intensively studied could accept or abandon the habit without withdrawal symptoms; none of them showed true physical dependence; none of them had shown a tendency to increase dosage, and most, when given as much as they asked for, tended to be quite moderate in their demands or to reduce dosage.[1]

The only reports of marihuana 'addiction' in Western society come from two groups of misfit American Army soldiers who seem to have been angling for discharges on the grounds of their drug use. Their cases are of some interest, because they illustrate vividly how even a drug that is agreed to have no physically addicting properties can nevertheless produce intense psychological dependence in personalities that suffer from sufficient social and psychological imbalance.

The two psychiatrists in charge of one group, mainly of coloured men, write:

Marihuana addicts are unaffected by social disapproval, rewards, punishments or any of the incentives or deprivations which affect the behaviour of normal or even neurotic patients. . . . A completely adequate estimate of the effects of marihuana can only be obtained by viewing its use as part of an entire life pattern. The problems of marhuana addiction cannot be understood from the study of its effects on non-addicts or on persons who do not become addicts – that is on persons to whom the personality problems of addiction are foreign. It needs to be emphasized that the problem is not the drug, but the users of the drug – the addict in relation to himself and society.

As a group their backgrounds were heavily loaded with adverse familial, social and economic factors. Their histories were characterized by delinquency and criminal behaviour and failure to develop any consistent life patterns of productive work. In fact, they felt and acted like enemy aliens towards society.

The personality picture of such addicts shows a typical response pattern to repeated situations of frustration and deprivation. This consists on the one hand of immediate and constant gratification of the need for sensual pleasure and for omnipotence, as well as the need to overcome their unbearable anxiety. On the other hand they show hostility and aggression towards others, especially those in authority, with the neurotic creation of situations that lead to further suffering. The addictive smoking of marihuana serves simultaneously as a satisfaction of all these drives. It is but one aspect of a complex picture of maladjustment.[18]

The most thorough investigation of the role of marihuana in normal society was done in New York at the instance of Mayor La Guardia, and published in 1944. Smoking was found mainly in Harlem and the Negro districts, happening in 'tea pads' – comfortable rooms with a juke box, dim lights and sexy pictures on the walls. 'The tea pad takes on the atmosphere of a very congenial social club. The smoker readily engages in conversation with strangers, discussing freely his pleasant reactions to the drug and philosophizing on subjects pertaining to life in a manner which at times appears to be out of keeping with his intellectual level.' It was found that smokers, unlike alcohol drinkers, know to a nicety how much they need to get 'high', and having reached that condition could not be persuaded to take more.

If a tea pad were shut, the disappointed smoker would go back to what he was doing – working or playing pool – perfectly calmly. This reaction contrasted so strikingly to that of heroin addicts cut off from the source of their drug, that the committee was convinced of the non-addictiveness of marihuana. It also found no connection between the drug and sexuality and crime, and no evidence that marihuana smoking leads to narcotic addiction.[19]

This report was a prime weapon of the 'doves' of the American drug control; it immediately drew a blast of fire from the former Commissioner Anslinger, a super-hawk in charge of the Federal Bureau of Narcotics, who is probably personally responsible by his rigidity for a good deal of America's present drug problem. In a style strikingly reminiscent of *Pravda*, he refers to

a very unfortunate report released some years ago by the so-called

La Guardia committee on marihuana. The [Federal] Bureau [of Narcotics] immediately detected the superficiality and hollowness of its findings and denounced it. However it gave wide circulation to the idea that this drug is relatively innocuous. The La Guardia report is the favourite reference of the proselytor for narcotic drug use.[20]

But he is unable to produce more than narrative evidence for his condemnation of marihuana and his contention that it leads inevitably to opiate addiction.

Even before the La Guardia Report the relationship between crime and marihuana had been exhaustively studied. A survey by the District Attorney of New Orleans found that in 1930, 125 out of 450 men convicted of major crimes were regular marihuana smokers. About half the murderers and a fifth of those convicted for assault, larceny and robbery were users.[21] Startling though these figures are, there is no attempt to claim that marihuana caused or facilitated these crimes, and they show no more than that in that society the people who commit violent crime also tend to smoke marihuana, probably both because of the same underlying psychopathy. A causal connection is denied in another investigation by the same writer of 17,000 felonies and 75,000 misdemeanours in New York City between 1932 and 1937: he found hardly any relation between serious crime and marihuana use, and no correlation at all with murder or sex crime.[22] This result was confirmed twenty-two years later in yet another study of 14,954 convictions in the New York County Court of General Sessions.[23]

As has now become well known, the American Army, the defender of the freedom of the West, is riddled with 'drug abusers'. In peaceful Europe large proportions of the American garrisons use marihuana in a more or less illicit way; while among combat troops in Vietnam, use of the drug was general and overt. So far no one has suggested that America's military reversals in that theatre were due to the pernicious effects of marihuana.

The same problems showed themselves recently in the British Forces, particularly the British Army on the Rhine, and all three services had, by early 1970, set up special drug squads. Drug abuse is apparently seen as being not only undesirable in terms of its ordinary effects, but also as exposing abusers to the risk of security blackmail.

In fact, in the psychiatric literature of European societies in the West it is difficult to find any convincing accounts of personal or social damage due to the drug. There are occasional descriptions of precipitated psychotic states, such as this from Anslinger, where, as well as being unbalanced, the subject was unused to the effects of the drug.

One summer evening Moses M. bought his first two marihuana cigarettes for twenty-five cents each. After smoking them he said, 'I felt just like I was flying.' Moses, crazed with marihuana, went through the window of his hotel room, dropped eighteen feet onto the roof of the garage next door in his bare feet, and then went through the window of K.'s room, crying, 'God told me to kill this man.' Seizing K. by the throat, Moses beat him to death with his fists, after which he broke a chair on his victim's head. Then screaming that he was pursued by Hitler, Moses went out through the window, and dropped his two-hundred-pound frame to the alley thirty feet below. In court Moses had no recollection of the killing and asserted, 'I didn't want to hurt him.' 'Twenty years,' said the Court.[20]

The chain of cause and effect was far from certain. 'Was he mad because of the drug, or did he use the drug because he was mad?' is a difficult question to answer. It is possible that marihuana, like heroin, barbiturate or amphetamines, is used by some people to stave off their own particular sort of madness.

The uncertain reality of the way the external world looks to the user jibes with the kinds of reality differences experienced by some schizoid personalities. Psychoanalytically, this could be interpreted as a problem of the user's narcissism and how its changes affect his ego. . . . Some users may begin taking marihuana as an unconscious attempt to cope with and perhaps curb a developing psychopathology.[24]

A survey of 1,200 Indian cannabis smokers and drinkers showed that although the drug attracts the mentally unstable, and that the neurotic would usually choose the stronger of the two preparations available while the non-neurotic chose the weaker, the rates for psychosis among users were not significantly different from that among the rest of the population.[25] Only 0·1 per cent of Israeli hashish smokers need psychiatric treatment – a proportion that seems very low compared with the usual rate for schizophrenia of 1 per cent. These and similar results seem to suggest that either the cannabis psychosis is very rare indeed, or that it substitutes for other forms of psychosis, or even that the drug is protecting its users from ordinary psychoses. Allentuck in a survey of institution and hospital inmates found 9 cases of psychosis in 77 marihuana users, but remarks that

a characteristic marihuana psychosis does not exist. Marihuana will not produce a psychosis *de novo* in a well integrated, stable person. . . . Should a psychosis be precipitated in an unstable personality it may last only a few hours or it may be continued a few weeks. It may be controlled by the withdrawal of the drug, and the administration of barbiturates. The psychic habituation to marihuana is not so strong as to tobacco or alcohol. . . . There is no evidence to suggest that the continued use of marihuana is a stepping-stone to the use of opiates. Prolonged use of the drug does not lead to mental, physical or moral degeneration, nor have we observed any permanent deleterious effects from its continued use.[26]

The more lurid accounts of criminality and psychosis due to the drug come from Africa and the Middle East; often they do not stand up to critical examination. Murphy, reviewing accounts of cannabis psychosis, finds few cases that can certainly be distinguished from schizophrenia, alcoholism, precipitated functional psychoses, manic depressive states, and, particularly in North Africa, the acute toxic states brought about by malnutrition and endemic infection.[1]

A recent account of cannabis-induced crime from the Professor of Psychiatry at Ibadan University says that half of those convicted of murder were long-term cannabis users, and so were two thirds of burglars, and a third of those convicted of assault, battery and sex offences against women. He says, interestingly, that cannabis use is found mainly in 'in-between' sub-groups, people half way between tribal society and Western-type living.[27] But before one can accept the implications of this sort of report, one would at least want to know whether these criminals differed in their use of the drug from other members of their social groups. Even then one would have no causal connection between cannabis and crime. It is as meaningful to say of British criminals that 99 per cent drink tea.

It is interesting that recent (1973) research has turned away from the search after facts – which are, in any case, pretty well understood – to a more polemic role. One notorious experiment, reported first in the *Daily Telegraph* (19 March 1971) rather than a scientific journal, was some work by a team led by Professor Paton, head of the Department of Pharmacology at Oxford. He reported that if mice were injected with T H C, the active constituent of cannabis, it accumulated in their body fat and foetuses were born deformed. Furthermore, the mice were killed by larger doses. It seemed impressive until the relationship of dose to body weight was analysed. It then turned out that while the normal, social use of T H C was about 2 microgrammes per gramme of body weight, the mice died from injected doses of 1,000 mcg. to 5,000 mcg. per gramme. It was as if a grown man had been injected with nearly a *pint* of pure T H C: death would not be surprising. The *Guardian* commented the next day that 'it was unclear whether mice shouldn't use cannabis, or professors shouldn't use mice'.

Another exercise, also reported in the *Daily Telegraph* (6 October 1971), was research by Dr. Cockett into young prisoners at Ashford Remand Centre, outside London. He found that three in five of those interviewed began drug-taking with cannabis, and that only one in five was a 'successful' pot smoker in the sense that they continued to smoke only cannabis. The implication of this research, that cannabis leads to hard drugs, is rather vitiated to the critical observer by the high degree of selection of the subject population.

On the other hand the American Department of Defense, forced to recognize that its conscript army contains a large number of drug users, has had to begin to investigate what impact this may have on its military effectiveness. Thus, a survey of 720 hashish users in the army in West Germany found that 300 were moderate users who consumed 10 to 12 gm. monthly, and showed no 'ostensible adverse effects'.[34] (See also the research into veteran heroin addicts, p. 34). One suspects that the U.S. Army, unable to eradicate the use of marihuana even with the powerful apparatus of surveillance and control that it can apply to its troops, is being forced to accept that the drug is essentially harmless and, for the sake of its own public relations, to acknowledge this. A recent review of two thousand papers on marihuana[35] concluded that 'Given that any drug in excess is dangerous, marihuana stands up at least as well, and in many ways better, than those two socially accepted drugs, nicotine and alcohol'.

A recent move in America has been to try to improve the acceptability of the drug to the capitalist system by demonstrating that it does not produce an 'amotivational syndrome' – i.e., smokers are just as grasping as anyone else. Thus, much of the statement of M. R. Aldrich of *Amorphia*, a group dedicated to legalizing marihuana in California, to the President's Committee on Marihuana and Drug Abuse, was devoted to this problem. And some workers have even gone so far as to set up a research microeconomy, in which young men, segregated from the world, 'work' at making stools for payment in tokens, while being forced to smoke THC cigarettes. The authors[36] found that moderate drug use didn't interfere much with the subjects' acquisitive instincts, and pointed out with pride, in support of this finding, that the young men had gone on strike half-way through for more payment for their participation in the programme. Just like any other well-adjusted trade unionists.

An authoritative laboratory experiment conducted by Dr J. H. Mendelson of Harvard for the U.S. Army in 1974, but not made public[38] until late 1975 – and then under protest – found that even heavy marihuana use did not impair the willingness of its subjects to work for money, nor did it upset their cognitive, neurological or testosterone functions. Some weight gain and impairment of lung function, due to the smoke rather than the drug, were found.

Marihuana Use in Britain

The character of the society in which marihuana is used is vitally important in predicting its effects on individuals. This is partly because of its quality of enhancing mood, and partly because it is a drug, like alcohol, that has to be 'learnt'. If there were no society of marihuana users, there would be no new users. Unlike the opiates or amphetamines, marihuana produces neither physical dependence nor immediately pleasant effects. Often the first half dozen experiments are frightening when they are not disappointing; there is no good reason in the drug itself why one should persevere with it. To make an expert, who enjoys smoking, there must be an active society of smokers who will welcome the novice and persuade him that the unpleasant sensations he first gets from the drug are in fact delightful and worth repeating. Even more important, they have to supply him with ideas with which to express what is happening to him under the drug; otherwise all is strange and confusing. Becker quotes a musician who was introduced to the drug by his colleagues; they got up on the stand and played the same tune for two hours:

'Anyway, when I saw that, it was too much. I knew I must be really high if anything like that could happen. See, and then they explained to me that it's what it did to you, you had a different sense of time and everything.'

. . . In every case in which use continued the user had acquired the necessary concepts with which to express to himself the fact that he was experiencing new sensations caused by the drug. . . In this way marihuana acquires meaning for the user as an object which can be used for pleasure.[28]

This learning process is relatively time-consuming. It is going to be difficult to go through with it unless the people about the novice allow him to meet smokers; he may even be distracted by more compelling pleasures. Bearing these points in mind, it is not surprising that one finds marihuana use where one does, in two isolated, uninvolved, self-contained sub-groups of society: West Indian immigrants, who brought the habit with them, and students, who learnt it, via the beats, from American Negroes. Among both groups there is the necessary amount of social interaction, isolation from the prejudices and business of the rest of society, and for many, enough leisure and boredom to make the habit worthwhile. An interview in the *Sunday Times* with one

Andrew Venn Mowat, 'one of the most articulate and experienced undergraduates on the Oxford drug "scene"', expresses these points clearly.

. . . 'pot' is an acquired taste. The first half dozen times were disappointing, but Oxford encouraged him in the habit. The University, he thinks, might almost be designed to nourish drug addiction. 'You've got this vast, amorphous amount of work that you more or less can or can't do as you wish. This and the permissive atmosphere about the place means that there's no real form to existence here. Marihuana gives it form. There's this part of the day when you know you'll be happy . . . You're free of the feeling – a common one in Oxford – that something marvellous is happening round the corner.'[29]

A recent study of student drug users in an English provincial university[32] found that the 'average student has taken a "soft" drug (especially cannabis) at least once without apparent effect on his career or personality, since there were no significant differences between the cannabis takers and a control sample in either university career or examination performance'.

Although cannabis has the reputation of being the favourite drug of the young, a survey in 1970 by the *Daily Mirror* found little to confirm this. It turned out that only 9 per cent of the sample, aged between 15 and 19, had ever tried pot (this would, if representative of the country at large, imply that 300,000 teenagers have used the drug once), and less than half had tried it again. More than three quarters thought that the drug should never be legalized, and only 18 per cent thought it should.[33] By 1973 rather more people had become familiar with the drug. A survey by the B.B.C.'s *Midweek* programme showed four million people had tried cannabis.[37]

My own first experience of hashish was with a group of Oxford derivation. I had been introduced to a number of smokers; they were friendly but guarded; until they had seen me using the drug I was not entirely to be trusted. They were intelligent, rather rebellious people, out of sympathy with the ordinary run of our society. Several of their parents had been refugees from Hitler's Germany, so perhaps they had better reasons than most for mistrusting the good intentions of their fellow men. One of them, an engineer who had served a three-month sentence for possession of marihuana, at length agreed to turn me on. He rang with the address – a narrow door beside a greengrocer's in Earls Court. We climbed five flights of stairs behind a small plump American girl called Johnny. The halls were dark, but under the door lights shone and there was a racket of many conversations. At the top she led us to a box room, tiny, furnished with a beat-up electric fire, an empty trunk, an iron bedstead with a theatrically grimy ticking mattress. On the wall someone had painfully pencilled

> Keep a clean nose
> Watch the plain clothes
> It don't take a weather man to
> Tell which way the wind blows.

My friend, a dark, nervous boy, arrived a few minutes later with the hash – a thumbnail-sized ball which he carefully broke and rolled into pellets. I don't normally smoke, so we were to balance these pellets on the glowing end of a lighted cigarette, and suck the smoke up through a Biro tube. 'Oh lovely!' exclaimed a deep-bosomed blonde. 'That's how they do in in Algerian prisons – only with a straw.' It seemed an ill-omened observation, but we went to work with a will. As guest, I was handed the tube first and bent over the ashtray. The smoke rose from the pellet in a thick column; when I sucked it bent over pleasingly and went up the Biro. But the lung pain was intense – I coughed like a jet engine lighting up and the precious pellet hurtled off into the dark. After a rest and a couple more tries and lost pellets I had acquired enough control to turn away before I exploded. By the time we'd used up all the pellets the boy who'd brought the stuff and Johnny were lying on the floor giggling, in the state known pleasantly to psychologists as 'fatuous euphoria' – either real or psychosomatic. I was hugging my agonized chest, and felt nothing else at all. So I went home to bed; by all accounts they had a thoroughly enjoyable evening.

Since then I have become slightly more expert; I can inhale without coughing every time. But on the other hand, the drug seems to have no strikingly noticeable effects. I have sometimes felt more giggly than usual, and enjoyed music more. The effect was much like that of a couple of stiff drinks, though without the blurriness of sensation that alcohol produces. On the other hand the impact of nicotine from the tobacco which is usually mixed with hashish or dried marihuana leaves to make a joint is most unpleasant. Normally I never smoke, and I find that within minutes of inhaling my limbs are tingling, I sweat all over, my heart pounds, I feel faint and nauseous. This passes within twenty minutes but often completely masks the pleasant effects, if any, of the cannabis.

8
Hallucinogens

The most hotly disputed illicit drugs are, for the moment, the hallucinogens. The buttons of the Mexican *peyotl* cactus have been used in that country since Aztec times; the principal active alkaloid, mescaline, was isolated and synthesized as 3,4,5-trimethoxyphenylethylamine in the twenties of this century. LSD-25, d-lysergic acid diethylamide, often inaccurately known as lysergic acid – a related substance with no interesting psychic effects – was synthesized in 1938 by Hofman in the Sandoz Laboratories at Basle; its psychic properties were noticed when he accidentally sniffed up a few microgrammes in 1943. It is now the most convenient and most used hallucinogen. A newer substance is psilocybin, the active principle in another Mexican plant, the sacred mushroom *Psilocybe Mexicana*. This was brought to the attention of the Western world in 1953 and also synthesized by Hofman. Less used drugs of the same general class are *ololiuqui*, the South American morning glory, *teonanacatl*, another Mexican mushroom that grows on cow-pats, *caapi*, an Amazonian vine, which is chemically identical with *yageine*, *harmine*, *banisterine*. *Bufotenin*, the venomous secretion of the skin of certain toads, has dramatic effects and is chemically identical to serotonin. The English hop plant is a type of morning glory, of which two varieties contain natural LSD, so it is not impossible that ordinary British beer has traces of hallucinogens.

LSD is now the most powerful mind-affecting substance known. Twenty microgrammes (a microgramme, 1 micg. or $\gamma = 0\cdot000001$ gramme) is enough to produce detectable effects and amounts to about 1/700,000,000 of a man's weight. As powder this quantity is almost invisible. Minute as such a dose is, an even smaller amount reaches the brain. Even when the ordinary dose of between 50 and 200 mcg. is taken, only 2/100 mcg. is available in the brain, or less than one molecule of LSD to every 3,000 brain cells.[1] More surprisingly, even this small amount has left the brain within twenty minutes of taking the drug, while the effects of the dose do not begin in less than thirty minutes to one hour, and last for four to eight hours. It is supposed, therefore, that the hallucinogens act as triggers, releasing some body chemical that produces the celebrated psychic effects.

The observable physical effects of LSD are slight. Goose-pimples, stronger tendon reflexes – the knee jerk, for example – and enlarged irises are the most noticeable. Less often the drug causes nausea and muscle pain, symptoms interpreted on no very good evidence by dynamic psychiatrists as mechanisms of defence against ego loss in unstable personalities. Neurologically, its effects are complicated. Although it inhibits signals in the optic nerves of cats, it also produces 'alerting cortical responses'[2] and lowers thresholds for vision and hearing. In general it hinders the transmission of signals across nerve synapses – the junctions of the brain's electrical circuits, and it also seems to break down the electrical insulation between neighbouring circuits so that signals can spread sideways. (A physical analogy for this 'mind enhancing' drug might be spraying salt water inside a television set.) This might account for the interesting effect called synaesthesia: the transference of impressions from one sense to another. Thus LSD subjects can hear hands clapping as showers of sparks, or feel a mild electric shock on the forearm as a bolt through the whole body. These phenomena seem to suggest that the drug breaks down the processes that limit and channel sense impressions in the deeper interpretative layers of the brain, allowing neuronal excitation to spread indiscriminately sideways. Curiously, although one of the commonest effects of the drug is the overwhelming impact of all sense impressions, it also appears to produce many of the signs of sensory deprivation.[3] This may be because it reduces the filtering effect of the outer layers of the brain and so effectively prevents any useful information getting through at all. One might compare the brain to an office organization that handles vast quantities of small pieces of information, at each level summarizing, correlating and passing on this material to the next level for action and further condensation.

Finally, the head of the organization – or the consciousness – is presented with one simple image. But LSD disrupts this delicate process; the millions of small messages pour straight through and completely swamp interpretation. Perhaps one could carry the analogy further, and say that the consciousness, in the manner of overworked executives, tends to seize at random on one or two messages and concentrates its attention on them, thus giving the impression of increased perception.

This interpretation of LSD's action is largely guesswork, but a pointer in the same direction is given by the research result that subjects already in an environment which deprives them of sense impressions – suspension in a tank of blood-hot water, for example – react less to LSD both psychologically and physiologically than they do when they are in the open, subjected to the normal barrage of stimuli.[1] It is also found that totally blind people, as opposed to those with even a little activity in the optic nerve, have no visual hallucinations.[4]

Although people under the influence of the drug often say that 'time has no meaning', or 'time stands still', when they are asked to guess at intervals between 15 and 240 seconds, they consistently call time *before* it is actually up. In other words intervals seem *longer* than they actually are, as they do when we are bored or understimulated.[3] This finding is curiously at odds with the riot of sense impressions some LSD subjects report, and again suggests that the drug interrupts sensory inputs that are in some way connected to our internal clock.

The subjective effects of LSD can be roughly summarized thus:
1. Sense impressions are perceived more strongly, colours are brighter, sounds like the ticking of clocks, that one would not normally listen to, become strikingly audible.
2. The mechanism that relates one sense impression to another is disabled, so that if a subject touches himself he may find it difficult to be sure that *his* hand is touching *his* leg, and vice versa.
3. The relationship between current sense impressions and past experience is knocked out, so that one sees things as it were for the first time. Aldous Huxley's ineffable garden chair in *The Doors of Perception* is a famous example.

4. Muscular coordination and pain perception are reduced.

5. Personality testing shows that learned patterns of behaviour, logical thinking, role playing, the elaborately acquired methods that enable us to survive and succeed, tend to be dissolved away.

6. With the eyes shut, swirling patterns of colours and shapes are seen.

7. Hallucinations, ranging from images known to be no more than fantasies to full-blown involvement in an unreal world, are common.

8. Emotional repressions are attacked, and one behaves, for better or for worse, more fundamentally. Emotional reserves between people under LSD are broken down, and they become more sensitive to each others' personalities.

9. Memories and experiences that have been severely repressed into the unconscious can be released and experienced as reality. In neurotics and psychotics this experience can be overwhelming and damaging.

So far, the effects of LSD can be summed up by saying that the drug dissolves the crust that separates us both from the sensually experienced world and our own unconscious. The effect on civilized man is often that he discovers – to his surprise – as large and strange a world inside his head as there is outside.

At this point it may be as well to mention two canards which have been spread about concerning LSD. The first is that American students who had taken LSD looked at the sun in a mystical trance and suffered retinal burns. This received world-wide publicity, but the correction issued by the Governor of Pennsylvania, that the story had been made up by the State's Commissioner for the Blind, who was himself blind, and at the time 'sick and distraught', has been less widely noticed.[9] The second is that LSD-taking causes damaged chromosomes. There have been a number of papers on this, and the general consensus seems to be that no such damage is found.[10]

The effects of LSD on personality are general, and vary with the individual; one of the few repeatable, measurable results claimed is a decreased performance on the Porteus Maze Test. In this, the subject is given a set of ten printed mazes graded from easy to almost impossible. He is given an unlimited number of attempts and unlimited time. The score, calculated from the difficulty of the last maze solved, number of tries and the time taken, measures social adaptation, forethought and self-control; it is claimed to be one of the very few tests that reliably distinguishes psychotics from normals.[5]

This leads us to the tantalizing connection between the LSD state and schizophrenia. For a while, after the war, it was thought that LSD produced in the normal investigator a 'model psychosis' that would be a great help in deciphering the puzzles of schizophrenia. Thus this class of drugs was given the name 'psychomemetic' – psychosis mimicking. But this idea has now been abandoned. The LSD state differs from the schizophrenic in several important points (see below), and it is now thought that the drug is no more than a useful training aid for psychiatrists who can get, with its use, something of the flavour of the world of schizophrenia. Often sufferers from this disease have said how refreshing and hopeful it is for them to talk to people who at least had some idea of what they experienced. The psychic similarity is paralleled by chemical likenesses, and the work of elucidating these clues has proceeded energetically since Osmond and Smythie's important paper in 1952[6] suggesting schizophrenia was caused by a breakdown in the body's capacity to handle adrenaline, a substance very similar to mescaline, and that therefore the body poisoned itself with a hallucinogen. In 1962 Friedhoff and Van Winkle[7] in New York isolated another mescaline relative, 3,4-dimethoxyphenylethylamine, from the urine of some schizophrenics, and this result has recently been confirmed by Clarke in Liverpool who, with a large sample and rigorous controls, recently found that 80 per cent of paranoids excrete this substance, while controls do not. But the chemical cure of schizophrenia is still a long way away.

LSD states also show interesting similarities with the experience of sensory-deprivation subjects and sufferers from delirium tremens. It is tempting to guess again that all four conditions are caused by the central consciousness' starvation of interpreted sense messages; into the vacuum flows unconscious material – electrical mid-brain activity that is usually suppressed by signals from outside and the brain's learned methods of dealing with them. One could make a crude analogy with the whispers of far-off, inane conversations one hears on trunk telephone calls over bad lines. But in the mind this buried activity that LSD and these other states uncover is far from inane. In the sick, the schizophrenic or the alcoholic, who are what they are partly because of their inability to adjust to themselves and their view of society, this material is often full of menace and dread, reflecting their destructive apprehension of the world and their place in it. The same thing sometimes happens when LSD is given therapeutically to neurotics. But often the healthy person, in a benign environment, finds this bathing in the raw world and his unconscious an exhilarating, even an exalting experience. Some would take it further, and make it the basis of new religions, or new approaches to old religious truths.

This table[8] summarizes some relationships between the LSD, schizophrenic, delirium tremens and sensory deprivation states.

	D.T.	Schizo-phrenia	Sensory deprivation	LSD
Perception				
Intensification of colour and depth	—	rare	+	+
Visual illusions	+	rare	+	+
Visual pseudo hallucinations	+	rare	+	+
Visual hallucinations	+	rare	+	+
More acute hearing	—	—	+	+
Auditory hallucinations	+	+	+	rare
Hallucinations of touch, taste and smell	rare	rare	+	rare
Emotions				
Euphoria	rare	rare	rare	+
Anxiety	+	+	+	+
Emotional instability	+	+	+	+
Inappropriateness of feeling	+	+	+	+

Body image	D.T.	Schizo-phrenia	Sensory deprivation	LSD
Feeling that self is unreal	+	+	+	+
Feeling that world is unreal	+	+	+	+
Ideation				
Fantasies	+	+	+	+
Flight of ideas	+	+	+	+
Feeling that neutral features of the world have a personal meaning	+	+	+	+
Delusions	+	+	+	+
Impairment of concentration	+	+	+	+
Impaired intelligence-test scores	+	+	+	+
Orientation				
Bad for time	+	+	+	+
Bad for place	+	+	+	+
Motor coordination				
Impaired	+	+	+	+

Inward Bound

The LSD experience differs from the other three described above in its potential beauty, and its power to bring over-civilized man into close and invigorating contact with his animality. An American philosophy student describes his supervised, experimental experience:

On the Rorschach I had great pleasure over the shadings on the plain black-and-white cards. The cards aroused my boundless admiration and I repeatedly said that I hadn't appreciated what a fine and intricate set of patterns they were. I was impressed with the effect of overprinting, where one pattern was placed on top of another one. As I associated to the cards, it was much the atmosphere of a dream. I was floating along with the reverie, not watching it from the shore. At intervals the door opening or a glance at myself would remind me that I was in an experiment, that I had had a drug, that this was a strange experience, but this was not disturbing, just on a par with the rest of my reverie. The coloured cards were magnificent. Each colour seemed to carry its own feeling tone, all positive. The oranges, reds and yellows were vital and expansive and sexual. The blues and greens were cool, serene and rational. I realized that normally I was a thinker more than a feeler and I revelled in the warmer shades which represented a release from obligation. But I didn't dislike the cool tones although I was aware that I couldn't think much now. It seemed to me that probably the rational activities were the better part, but the sensuous qualities of colour and tension and activity were attractive and engrossing now. I reflected several times that I was giving much the same interpretations I had some years earlier, the same volcanoes, the same sexual symbols – only they were franker this time, the same restless and powerful animals, but I wasn't a bit unhappy about this. Rather I admired the intensity of images, the aliveness of the figures, without concern about the interpretation the psychologist would put upon these responses. . . .

Some time after the Rorschach, it was suggested we go for lunch. The hall seemed lovely and impressive and I remember remarking that it was quite a contrast to the drab hall I had seen on entering; then it occurred to me that this might not be a polite way to refer to their building. But I felt they wouldn't mind, after all it wasn't their responsibility the way the place was decorated. My face was quite flushed and I looked tousled and it must have been apparent to many that I was a patient or a subject. When I noticed an attendant or nurse looking at me curiously, I would momentarily think 'I must look very odd'. Normally I would be quite embarrassed at such attention, but I didn't mind it at all. Rather, I felt a warm affection for anyone interested in looking at me curiously. The canteen appeared as a beautiful and most attractive hall peopled by the loveliest of characters and filled with the most dazzling food. The salads, the meat balls, the vegetables, all were gloriously radiant.

Some days later he wrote:

The most impressive characteristic of the experience was an enormous and, for me, unique sense of freedom. Normally I am unconscious of the tension and strain under which I live, but the difference between my usual state and the one I enjoyed during this experience is so great that it could be compared to the lifting of a heavy burden.

Another subject, a young psychiatrist who seems to have borne his obligations rather heavily, felt that whatever LSD's effects he ought to remember his professional dignity, and said afterwards,

Somehow I was rather surprised when I found out under lysergic acid I was really rather a nice, warm sort of person. The other feeling I retain is that no matter how bad things get I always have a nice, comfortable, warm place to go. The feeling is almost as if I carried a quiet, pleasant, serene garden around in my head.[1]

Experiences on the LSD trip are extremely unpredictable, and vary with the same individual from occasion to occasion. My own essay took me neither to grandeur nor horror; it is perhaps typical of many that are not otherwise thought worth writing up.

A big, bare, white room in Paddington. The mantelpiece is hidden by blow-ups of photographs taken by the owner, a nervous Australian pot-smoker. His round-headed friend sits like a wooden doll on the floor – a long way away from us. He says, 'It's incredible here, man, everyone's on the LSD kick.' His remark had nothing to do with the conversation; he spoke slowly, as if he weren't thinking exactly of the same things that you were, or even anything like them; as if he were holding another, silent, conversation in between the gaps of your own. I said I was interested in the stuff, and he looked arch: 'Perhaps I should make you a proposition.' I gave him thirty shillings and he went up the road for ten minutes, came back and sat down, looking straight in front of him as though he had not moved. Half an hour later, I made to go. He pulled a small silver cube from his pocket: 'Do it with someone you like – and have your wife handy,' he said, as though these might be two distinct people. In my case, it's the same person. As we were going to bed – because of looking after the children during the day I'd thought it would be best to take the LSD experience at night – she hadn't been keen to try. Then, as we were getting undressed, she said yes. I got a black plastic plate and a knife, and cautiously cut the corner off the sugar cube. We split it, and ate; I expected Hofman's first instant reaction. Of course, nothing. After half an hour, we ate the rest, made some self-pitying jokes about buying sugar at £300 a box and went to bed.

The trouble was that we couldn't sleep. At first I thought it was being excited, and anyway there was a full moon which always keeps me awake. Then after an hour, Barbara said she could see patterns. Sick of lying still, I went downstairs to get some paper and a pencil. I picked up a pink Biro: suddenly, there it was – the pinkness, the huge hand, the fleshness. 'It works, it works, come out in the light,' I yelled up the stairs.

We turned on the bedroom light and waited for visions. All

that happened at first was that the room looked less white, colder and crooked. It is in fact white all over with a pleasant fluted wallpaper put in by the interior decorator who had it before us, with heavy white Victorian cornices and white blinds. Normally it's a pleasant, soft, diffuse box for sleeping in. The walls weren't pure white any more – yellowish. But I began to think the hand bit downstairs meant nothing. I picked up a box of little disk magnets the children had been given; there was a tube of iron filings with them. If you poured the filings on the magnets, they clustered furry and curved in on themselves, they looked like space monsters. As you pulled the two disks apart the filings stretched out in knobbly arms, then fell back like the petals of a flower. When they came together again the petals reached out to each other, and near enough they stroked each other, some petals growing longer by the contact. We could hear the rustle of the filings over each other as the moving magnetic fields re-arranged them.

I felt things were beginning to look odd, but only out of the corners of my eyes. If I glared, they immediately looked all right. Then I scratched the back of my head. This definitely was odd. There was a tremendous noise of threshing wheatfields. I could feel hair roots bending, knotting the scalp. There were the feelings a field gets being harrowed – by my finger-nails I supposed. I was fairly sure someone was scratching someone's head, and that someone's head seemed to be being scratched; but it was difficult to be sure whose or by whom.

It was as if inside one's head there were an alert observer, who at moments like this would have said: 'The scratching sensations from fingers and scalp correlate with your arm and head positions: you are scratching your head.' The drug had retired him; I had to solve the problem by sheer intellectual effort. My children, when they were small, used to reach up, grasp an ear, then they would burst into tears because someone was pulling it. Suddenly I could understand their predicament.

Barbara was holding her left arm before her face. 'It's like an old film; it lurches,' though she was holding it still. I tried with a hand, and it writhed slowly like the tentacles of a sea anemone (apparently the eyeball wriggles all the time to shift images on to fresh bits of retina; this movement is invisible until L S D knocks out the compensating mechanism, so one sees things moving slowly). It had taken quite a long time to get this far – the use of the word 'trip' for an L S D experience is quite appropriate, though not in the sense one might imagine of strange lands and romantic experiences. For us it was very like going on a modern journey by aeroplane, say: a little fear, homely surroundings, aches, staying awake all night, dirtiness, more fear, the flat garish light of indoors at four in the morning. I became conscious of how badly made the house was; each particle of dust on the floor stood out like an overdone T V commercial for sink washing-powder. Colours were richer – the old varnished floorboards escalated from being just old varnished boards to a rich, cynical *House and Garden* honey colour, but the effect wasn't particularly pleasant.

It began to feel irritating with the light on, like being at a fun fair too long, so we turned it out and tried to go to sleep. In some ways this was a mistake. Barbara began to mutter about the colours she could see: mauves and oranges – 'There it goes – a lovely purple.' She enjoyed this bit; for a long time I could see no patterns and felt cheated, then suddenly I was inside the hollow tooth of a lobster, with a fine view out of his mouth at an army of handsome buff-coloured legs walking along beside us. When he ate, the noise was enormous, like a giant eating lettuce. Then I was Low's T.U.C. horse, covered in buff nylon fur, with five legs and having a shoe nailed inside my mouth. Neither of these illusions, though vivid, was alarming. Then the patterns began: a line of lights so bright I looked round the room to see what they were. They grew into dots and dashes, squares, cubes and little balls all intricately packed and dissolving together. Barbara began to say: 'Oh hell, this is agony. When will it stop. What a ghastly life people must lead who take this for fun.'

Lying still became impossible because of the contact of clothes or each other. My left arm felt horrible – light and infuriating. I wanted to tear it off and have some peace. One's mind's eye kept sinking and swooping, dashing about and dissolving into itself,

117

creating mad situations and simultaneously chopping and serving them a dozen at a time; the whole process ticking onwards in jumps like a metronome.

Sounds became clearer – we could clearly hear someone winding up a watch next door; and we could hear every breath of a strange baby crying in some house down the street. Barbara seemed to sleep, then sat up, looked about her carefully, and said: 'How many pairs of gloves am I?' She said afterwards that she'd been standing in High Street, Kensington, wondering who she was; she'd had to make an inventory round the room: 'Who do I know who owns that pair of shoes, that dress? It must be Barbara Laurie.'

Although I felt so odd, I found I could write legibly, and wrote down some fairly full notes. Thinking about it afterwards, it seems obvious that we had split a fairly small dose; anything larger would have precluded note-taking. Just as well. We could see very clearly the predicament we were in, like travellers stranded in some bizarre place. Often it seemed funny. We had been some months before to see 'Villa 21', a free-range unit for young schizophrenics in a mental hospital to the north of London. Barbara said now: 'Someone, somewhere, must be able to make sense of all this,' and we both giggled nervously, because one of the boys there had sat about conspicuously saying: 'What's the meaning of it all? Someone must know?'

We turned the light off again. I began to feel frighteningly sure that this was madness; being roller-coastered inside your own head, knowing it was all illusion, yet unable to stop or control it. Time went unbearably slowly, and often seemed to slip backwards, so that the precious five minutes won towards release would slither away again in a whirl of sparks. I thought of the plight of madmen in their narrow hospital beds, with not just the problem of winning through until morning, when it would all – I sincerely hoped – go away, but through tomorrow and tomorrow and the next day and the next night, until when? Worse than a prison sentence because you would have no peace. It was like being locked up in a little-ease with a lunatic who wouldn't stop letting off fireworks.

We had sex – you couldn't call it making love – for something to do. At least it felt fairly normal, though towards the end I was in a church crypt where invisible craftsmen were gilding choir stalls; Barbara had something to do with a lot of Moroccan handbags. It was meagre on sensation, and as we stopped the patterns began again, I found I could smell now: with a little practice I could distinguish the smell of my left armpit from my right and each finger had a different, rich, gamey scent. Our two-year-old daughter, who is very fat and self-confident, came into the bed for a while. We both clung to her because she was so sane and normal. Barbara made us laugh by sitting up and theatrically declaiming: 'So onward they slept, wearily gnashing their multi-coloured teeth.' She drifted off to sleep, and dreamt that the iron filings were cream she had to swallow, and were coagulating in her throat; then later about two unhealed burns on her finger: she could see into the red pit, right into the cell structure and the quivering walls of proto-plasm.

The next day we felt cold and remote, but got through a lot of work. Driving the children to school, I nearly crashed when a coloured girl came out of a grey house wearing day-glo orange trousers: they went off on my retina like a bomb in a free-church assembly. It is difficult to explain how long and gritty and un-satisfying the LSD experience was. For several months we used it as a comparison for anything unpleasant; yet the results were not at all bad. We both felt that it made us more sensitive to shape and colour, and that it made us more dispassionate about other experiences and relationships, more direct about our day-to-day intentions. None of these effects was profound, but LSD seemed to jolt us forward over a stretch of maturing we'd probably have covered anyway. Like a tough expedition, one came away from it saying, 'If I can cope with that, I can cope with a lot of other things too.' One thing I couldn't have got another way was an understanding of the tenuous links between the outside world, my own past experiences and my consciousness. Before this trip I had made several attempts to read Laing's *The Divided Self*, an analysis of a certain type of schizophrenia, without being able to get any sense from it; afterwards it read like a guide-book to the town of my birth. For us the LSD experience was less important than the carpets it lifted and the structure of our minds we saw below.

9
LSD Applied

'A lump of sugar with two small dark stains, but it can be all of heaven and all hell to some poor bastard after he sucks it.'

Cassandra, *Daily Mirror*, 4 April 1966

In the first fine flush of enthusiasm after the war between the fifties and the sixties, L S D was acclaimed as a psychotherapeutic wonder drug. In Canada, for example, it was used extensively for the treatment of acute alcoholics. Under one régime, they were, on 'Truth Day', given massive, 400 mcg. doses in the hope that they would suffer an experience so profound and shattering that it would change the entire course of their life. For a while, as with every new psychiatric method, successes were reported, but as it became routine, and the real factor in treatment, the interest and enthusiasm of the therapists, waned, so results fell away. After three and a half years none of a representative group who had been given L S D had stopped drinking, and indeed showed hardly any improvement.[1]

In the same way a group of prisoners treated with psilocybin by Leary and his colleagues did indeed show some improvement, and for a short time after their discharge were jailed less often than one would expect. But how much this was due to the drug and how much to the researcher's contact, interest and effort to find the men houses and jobs, is extremely debatable.[2]

It is still used in psychotherapy by a very small number of English psychiatrists; a few more who might like to use it probably do not for fear of a mishap and possible scandal. It is interesting that one of those who does use it is a Jungian; his patients see visions of ancient Egypt and archetypal snakes.* One of his patient's experiences has become a classic in the literature of

---

*In the same way Hofman, when he experimented with synthesized psilocybin, knowing its derivation from mushrooms used in Aztec religious rites, saw his assistants with bronzed skins and high cheekbones, and thought that his laboratory was decorated with Mexican motifs.

hallucinogens. It vividly illustrates the drug's ability to bring back to consciousness repressed and troublesome memories, and to break up the tarmac-like coating that holds down these boiling forces. This woman, who at twenty-nine felt dead, lifeless, useless, had a fortnight's course of LSD. During that time she became again a child of six. She experienced her house during the day as her old school, with her children as her playmates; at night it was her childhood home. She felt child-size again; when she held her doctor's hand, it enveloped hers, she felt her clothes hanging about her in swathes.

I had the sensation as in my first LSD treatment of a snake curling up round me. I felt very sick and dizzy. Then I began to see serpents' faces all over the wall – then I saw myself as a fat pot-bellied snake slithering gaily away to destruction. I felt horrified and thought: 'Whose destruction?' I then realized that it was my own destruction, I was destroying myself. I seemed to be having a battle between life and death – it was a terrible struggle, but life won. I then saw myself on the treadmill of life – a huge wheel was going round and round with hundreds of people on it. Some were on top going confidently through life, others were getting jostled and trodden on but still struggling to go on living (I saw myself as one of these people), and then there were others who just couldn't cope with life and were being crushed to death in the wheel. I had another realization of how I was destroying myself – by carrying on this affair with this married man.... The doctor came in and asked me how I felt and I told him that there were snakes everywhere. I had the sensation of being right in the middle of them. The doctor asked me if it was like anything I had experienced before. I said it was a dream I had had as a child. He asked me if I knew what that dream represented and I said 'Sex'... I could see snakes slithering through the grass. The whole atmosphere was as it had been when sexual incidents occurred with boys when I was about six or seven.... I had a vision of life as a dark and murky pool and saw myself dipping my toes in gingerly with first one man and then with another, of being urged on by some of them to go down into the pool with them but I kept drawing back – I just had to wait for the right man to experience the pool of life with.

At the climax of the treatment she remembered a series of sexual assaults made on her during her childhood; even seeing the floor of the treatment room carpeted with the flowers and grasses of the wood where it happened.

Another woman who had always had 'something lacking in my life, no spark, a feeling of not really being here, incomplete', found herself, eventually, under L S D.

... inside a cell of my subconscious mind. It contained a spider, no longer alert and frightening and vivid, but tired, beaten and almost dead, it looked pathetic. With the spider there were thoughts and feelings and from these the conscious person, myself, sitting on the bed, had to learn a lesson. It was a most peculiar sensation. I found that my conscious self A was speaking to my subconscious self B. A was learning and speaking the lesson, B was teaching it by sending out waves of thought and feelings. A spoke the following words: 'The love I felt' – at this B sent a wave of pure love flowing through my body – 'The tears I shed' – a strong feeling of emotion came to my throat and tears to my eyes – 'the pain' – with this a terrifying weight on my body. At this point I got confused ... Eventually I cried because I was unable to understand and learn my lesson. I came out of my subconscious and sat on the bed thinking about what had just happened. I realized that I had been in the cell of memory containing my mother's death, that in it were the mistakes I had made at that time and from it I could learn a very valuable lesson.[3]

The therapist comments that 'L S D gives these people [obsessional neurotics and depressives] some real and tangible experience of their own unconscious and rekindles their faith in their own spirit.' However it is uncertain how much success is due to the drug, and how much due to the psychiatrist's preference for working with patients in this condition. The drug may facilitate his ability to cope with the patient as much as it enables the patient to cope with herself.

Again, the first enthusiasm for the drug as a cure-all having subsided, its use is restricted to fairly small classes of patients. Cohen gives this list of suitable cases for treatment:

people suffering from an excessively strict conscience, those who have lost confidence and self-esteem, those who are unable to overcome the grief of a personal loss. Depressions due to the environment, lost people who can find no meaning in existence, people with anxiety, passivity or aggression.

But he points out that L S D does no more than break down the mind's long-established defences to let the conscious see the unconscious; there still remains a long period of re-education before the patient can be said to be cured. L S D can only be a road breaker, and the changes it causes in ordinary personalities can only be at a shallow level: 'It is agreed that short-term therapy with L S D is a "super-ego cure" and that it changes only the attitudes and values of the patient' – not what he does with them.[4]

He gives as poor prospects: the eternal adolescent, the extremely depressed, the hysteric or paranoid – who may become convinced of his actual instead of only suspected god-head. The schizophrenic's symptoms are exacerbated by L S D, and the borderline schizophrenic may well be tipped over the edge. But these are hardly definite rules. Another English therapist had a young schizophrenic who felt he had died at the age of twelve; on his twenty-fifth birthday he was going to kill himself. He had been unsuccessfully in analysis for two years. On the eve of the birthday, he was given a large dose of L S D. There was a danger that he might kill himself, but he was determined to anyway. Instead, the next morning, he came in complaining that he should have had the drug years ago.

But the unwritten history of L S D therapy must contain many episodes like this: the patient showed chronic anxiety in a schizoid personality, he had been in analysis unsuccessfully, so he was given 25 mcg. of L S D. 'During the next few hours the patient kept repeating, "I see it all now," but refused to communicate with the therapist. Three days later he scratched his wrists with a razor blade. The depression lifted slowly, and he was eventually discharged from the hospital essentially unimproved.'[5]

The dangers to be expected from L S D are real. They are: personality change, prolonged hallucinations, psychosis, attempted suicide, addiction, poisoning, successful suicide.

Generally, these problems depend on the subject's previous instability, intensified by unfavourable surroundings during the drug experience. Personality change is, after all, one of the principal reasons for taking LSD. Mature, well-organized people who have had the drug claim in general that they are the better for it, they are more realistic in their relationships, more perceptive and mature.[2] Attitude tests on other samples show a general decrease in dogmatism and a greater tolerance for opposing views, and with anxious people, more peace of mind. The effect of LSD is on the most superficial level and it leaves the bedrock of personality undisturbed. People who show sudden reversals of character when taking the drug under good conditions are probably like those who suffer sudden religious conversions whose psychic forces were in precarious equilibrium.

One result of taking LSD repeatedly – about once a week – is that it seems in some people to produce a state of permanent cheerful carelessness.

The euphoria and detachment that so commonly follow frequent use of the drug seem to be habit [sic] to people who take drugs every week or two. The person who shows this euphoria as a result of repeated use of the drug may intellectually anticipate future problems but not be sufficiently concerned about them to act on the information. To the observer it seems that the drug experience sufficiently reduces general anxiety and customary learned unconscious defence mechanisms to require conscious defence [also sic]. It is as though the drug dissolved both realistic and neurotic fear and anxiety of life. The subject considers this general effect valuable because the majority of life's anticipated dangers and perplexities never materialize. He consequently feels safe and much more free from anxiety; indeed he may feel actually euphoric. Unfortunately when real trouble comes along, he may be too detached to act in what an outside observer would see as his best interests.[6]

The behaviour of the American LSD proselytizers seems to bear out this idea: one man was recently sentenced to a very considerable term of imprisonment in connection with the smuggling of half an ounce of marihuana through the American customs; five weeks after this sentence his house was raided and more marihuana was found there.[7] But one wonders how much this is the effect of the drug, and how much the behaviour of a personality that would rather be free of self-preserving fears – even

of a personality that shows the self-destructiveness very characteristic of people dependent on other drugs. This type of behaviour
is by no means confined to LSD users. When Christ asked his
disciples, 'Is not the life more than meat and the body than
raiment? Behold the fowls of the air. . . . Take therefore no
thought for the morrow. . . .'[8] their relatives may have been equally
alarmed at their euphoria and detachment. Before one blames the
drug for the more modern situation, one must ask also about the
personality that is willing to take the drug once a week for long
periods. It does not seem to be a common reaction; I certainly
would rather do anything but, and even those who have had
ecstatic experiences are not always willing to repeat them. One of
Cohen's subjects who had had the 'most blissful' experience said,
when he was offered another dose,

> I don't think that I will take the drug again, at least not now . . . I've
> had one wonderful day. Maybe we shouldn't ask for more than one
> such day in a life-time.[4]

Even more perhaps than other drugs, the situation in which
LSD is taken profoundly affects the subject's experience. When
one gets, as in America, serious, intellectual, rebellious people
using the drug as the foundation of an in-group rather similar in
atmosphere to a closed religious sect, it is going to be difficult to
distinguish drug and social effects from each other, or to decide
which are undesirable.

A more common problem in England, where LSD use seems
not to be so well organized as among some groups in America, is
going to be the impact of adverse surroundings on the drug
experience. The illicit user is unlikely to take the drug in the
company of people who understand what is happening to him
and are willing to reassure him about it. It is as if someone
dressed him in a diving suit and threw him into deep water without telling him how to work the valves. Even in clinical settings
the outcome of the drug experience can be uncertain.

If LSD is given under disinterested laboratory conditions while
impersonal assistants attach electrodes, take blood samples and perform
a number of other puzzling tasks, and if the subject gets the impression

that he will be temporarily mad and observers provide neither support nor reassurances, a psychotic state is bound to occur.[4]

Another researcher, writing of clinical applications of LSD:

It would probably be fairly easy to induce psychotic-like behaviour if subjects were put into a more stressful situation and made to feel more insecure.[9]

As if to prove his point, an associate soon after stole and took in secret 200 mcg. of LSD; it took two years to cure him of the resulting psychosis. It is probable that many people who have trouble after illicit use of hallucinogens resemble the case of a twenty-year-old American girl student who ate 250 morning glory seeds and went to hospital weeping, dissociated, saying she thought she would lose her mind. She had no hallucinations, and the effects were over in six hours. The psychiatrist who examined her comments that she had a 'hysteroid personality with deep, unsatisfied, dependent needs. Although insisting that she took the morning glory seeds out of sheer boredom, it is notable that this episode rallied divorced parents to her support.'[10]

It is probable that illicit LSD use is particularly attractive to intelligent, artistic, disorganized people whom one cannot call mad, but who nevertheless hardly connect properly with ordinary society. One such is a bohemian American female artist who had been in hospital five years before for dissociation, and after a dozen LSD experiences set off for Mexico to join a freedom group, but before she arrived it had disbanded. Her hallucinations were of curtains of light in front of her eyes, of people decomposing in the street, and lasted for five months after her last dose.

One of the tragedies reported in the literature is this, often quoted in opposition to illicit use of hallucinogens:

A twenty-four-year-old student chewed 300 (morning glory) seeds, equivalent to 300 mcg. LSD, had full-blown hallucinations and fantasies of saving the world, which lasted twenty-four hours even with sedatives. Mild exhilaration lasted for three weeks, when the hallucinations started again. Everything had double meanings, there was a ringing in his ears as in the drug intoxication state. He was afraid he was going insane, and needed sedatives again. Weeks later, he woke up one morning, was very upset because he thought he was out of balance again, drove his car down a hill and crashed into a house at 100 m.p.h.[11] Unfortunately we know nothing of his previous psychiatric history.

There is a growing international literature of LSD disasters – a recent murder in America, a Swiss doctor who ecstatically jumped in a lake and nearly drowned, a Scandinavian woman who went out and stabbed her seducer. A twenty-year-old English musician with no history of mental illness or instability took some LSD alone in his attic room. He locked himself in, scattered everything he possessed, broke the gas stove, the electric light fittings, all the windows and hurled himself off the roof. He fell four storeys onto a brick wall and was killed. Another young man, a bricklayer's labourer, again with no previous history of mental illness, seems to have gone to a club in Soho, where he was given LSD. Then he got to Highgate, some six miles away, climbed a church, took off his clothes, folded them neatly and jumped sixty feet to his death. Bewley comments: 'Despite the statements of the protagonists of this drug that it is safe, LSD can be dangerous when taken casually.'[21] In 1967 England had its first murder under the influence of LSD. An American, of the psychedelic sort, strangled an eighteen-year-old prostitute while they were making love: at the trial he said that because of the drug he thought she was a serpent and had defended himself. Because he lacked the intention to kill necessary for a conviction of murder, he was convicted of manslaughter and was sentenced to eight years' imprisonment.

The Advisory Committee on Drug Dependence report that 'Harmful mental states can occur. During the first few hours after taking the drug there may be violent behaviour, a panic-stricken or paranoid patient may attack others or he may hurt himself.' Some users had attempted to kill, or had in fact killed themselves or others, 'because they have apparently developed either a self-hatred or a feeling of superior power and invulnerability . . .'[22]

But alarming as these events are, it seems they happen rarely in comparison with the enormous number of licit and illicit LSD experiences in the Western world. A review of 25,000 reported administrations of LSD to 5,000 people found that among normals chosen for laboratory experiments, hallucinations lasting more than forty-eight hours occurred in 0·08 per cent of cases, and that none of these committed or attempted suicide. Among mentally disturbed patients who were given LSD in therapy, 0·18 per cent had longer than forty-eight-hour experiences, 0·12 per cent attempted suicide, and 0·04 per cent succeeded in killing themselves. Often suicide was many weeks later, in the patient's deep disappointment at the drug's failure to cure him.[12]

The authors of this paper comment, elsewhere,

> It is surprising that such a profound psychological experience leaves adverse residuals so rarely. This may lend support to the impression that psychological homeostatic mechanisms for handling acute stresses are more resilient than is commonly believed.[13]

A survey of the case papers of 67 people admitted to mental hospitals in Britain during 1966–7 who had used LSD, showed that 26 had had acute psychotic reactions – most of them found raving in public places – two had tried to commit suicide, three had made aggressive attacks on others, and there was nothing to show that the drug had had any effect on the other 36.[23]

Another review of a large number of LSD administrations showed that it was possible to predict untoward effects on the basis of short interviews before the drug was given. A typical paranoid reaction was shown by a twenty-eight-year-old married man who had complained in the interview that office cliques were plotting against him, refusing him promotion by advancing their own members. He felt that his immediate supervisor was harsh and unfair. He insisted that he was going to be given the largest dose of LSD. After taking the same amount as other subjects, he was surly and uncooperative, glared at everyone, and was cryptic and evasive in his answers to questions. The next day he described the plot he had seen among the other subjects and the experimenters, who wanted to take over the world. One of the doctors, wearing a goatee beard and a Martian uniform, was the master mind. Under the drug, he could tell the members of the conspiracy by the lines on their faces. He felt that the food he had been offered was poisoned, and he heard what is rare in LSD states, voices telling him to 'stay in line'. Remnants of this scheme of delusions stayed in his mind for two days after the experience.[14]

To recapitulate: the literature suggests that when LSD is given in proper conditions only those who are already detectably unstable are likely to suffer. Even without weeding, the risks of serious schizophrenic breaks or suicide are likely to be slight – no more than the risks we accept in everyday life or in many sports. In illicit use the drug is likely to be dangerous because unstable people are attracted to it, and their experiences are liable to produce unconscious guilts and fears they cannot handle alone. Cohen and Ditman report that the majority of paranoid reactions are found in people who got the drug on the black market.

Curiously, Cohen suggests that people who *give* LSD under poor conditions are likely to suffer more than the recipients:

After intensive, though sometimes only after brief, contact with the drugs, a few [therapists] have gone on to a psychotic breakdown or megalomaniac ideas of grandeur. Marked depressions in which these agents played a role are known. A couple of practitioners have found themselves in legal difficulties (this was before LSD as such was illegal in the U.S.A.) because of anti-social practices. This is an impressive morbidity, especially in view of the relatively small numbers of American practitioners using the hallucinogens.[4]

An English psychiatrist who used LSD intensively has given it up partly because 'giving the drug responsibly is even more demanding than taking it.'[15]

The risk of physical addiction to the drug is non-existent. This was demonstrated by an extremely careful experiment at Lexington, in which a group of Negro morphine ex-addicts – who were matched to controls outside the prison for sensitivity to LSD – were given mounting doses over a period of three weeks. After the first few days the hallucinations, delusions and confusion they experienced at first had gone, and by the end of this period almost all physiological signs of the drug's action had vanished. At the end they were being given 180 mcg. a day, in a glass of water; on the last day they were unaware that their dose was any more than water. Within three days their sensitivity to LSD was re-established. One subject was then given the 180 mcg. he had taken with equanimity before: 'he was very anxious, felt he was being shocked electrically, he felt that his body shrank and swelled, that his hands had extra fingers, that the walls were a mass of flickering colours, that he would die or become insane.'[16]

That is, although the effects of both LSD and heroin decrease with time, with LSD it is impossible to re-establish them by taking more; the body becomes completely insensitive to the drug, and there is no incentive for physical addiction in the ordinary sense.

This result, however, does not preclude the possibility of habituation. This state seems to differ slightly from habituation to other drugs, since it is rare for people to take it more than twice a week – more frequent dosage is made ineffective by de-sensitization – and the LSD state is chosen as an experience preferable, rather than as an alteration, to ordinary consciousness.

In man LSD has not been found to be toxic. Doses of 1,500 mcg. have been taken safely, though the effects are not pleasant. In animals death is due to respiratory paralysis, and in comparison to man even more gigantic doses are needed.[17] In one of the most expensive animal experiments ever performed, a group of Americans killed a borrowed circus elephant with LSD. Children, however, seem very sensitive to the drug, partly because their body weight can be three or four times less than an adult's, and therefore the relative dose is increased by that factor. As this is written, a five-year-old American girl is in hospital with suspected brain damage after eating a 50-mcg. LSD sugar lump she found in her parents' refrigerator.

Illicit Use of LSD

LSD is not only man's most powerful drug, it is the only one illicitly used that can be made informally in the United Kingdom. Heroin needs morphine or poppy from Asia; marihuana can be grown under glass, but it has the lack of flavour characteristic of forced vegetables. LSD can be made without much difficulty from the lysergic acid base; this in turn can be bought from chemical suppliers. If it cannot be bought, lysergic acid can be synthesized by an expert organic chemist who has time and equipment to devote to the problem. Since LSD at £1.50 a dose fetches about 600 times the cost of the commercial base, this synthesis might be attractive and feasible for a well-organized black-market operation. In certain circumstances, as the law stands, this manufacture and subsequent use would be legal. If the strong demand for it continues, it will be almost impossible to control the drug, for not only can it be made easily, it is even simpler to hide or import. The implications of these facts are discussed below in Chapter 11.

The illicit use of LSD is fairly new in Britain, and it is difficult to distinguish a pattern. So far it seems to be used in the same circles as marihuana, mainly among students who are fascinated by the emotional, intellectual and artistic implications of the drug; and as a supplement by the floating, beatnik, pan-addict populations of London, Bristol and Edinburgh. The B.B.C. *Midweek* survey showed that by 1973 650,000 people had tried LSD.[24]

This is the statement of a twenty-five-year-old sculptor, who was living with his parents in an immaculate semi-detached house in a London suburb when I interviewed him. 'This place is so sterile. I'd been six months sculpting in London, then I tried it in Bristol where there's a great drugs scene. But they're just a little gang of layabouts who hang out in this café with a pin-table and a Negro chewing gum – it looked so like an American documentary, it made you laugh. There was just one guy there, Steve, a seventh son of a seventh son who just radiated. You know, everything lit up when he came in. But it was so dull, I came home. I'll get a job this summer on the Dungeness nuke [the nuclear power station] labouring. I'll earn £33 a week; that'll set me up for the summer.'

He is tall, well-built, red-faced. He wears an eye-concussing shirt in prussian blue with orange and vermilion flowers. After my own LSD experience the shirt alone proclaimed the drug. His fingers too are smooth and pink and wave about like anemones.

He is talkative, and very uninterested in anything outside himself; his hair is curly and rises at the back in the way mod boys used to brush their beehives a year or so ago. There is something strikingly L S D about the whole of him, deep crude colours, writhing outlines like a vivacious *jugendstil* painting.

'I had four years at a provincial art school, a year at the one in Berlin. That was such a fantastic scene, it was worth ten. The trouble is I get hung up on teaching – you know, one day a week like most people do. But there's no point being poor so I earn money. After a bit you begin to appreciate the things money buys so you just automatically need more money. I don't really cop society. I mean, just look what they've done to Britain in the last fifty years. It's so ugly. The manifestations of our culture are hardly desirable.' We look out of his bedroom window at the carpet of semi-detacheds rolling over the downs.

'I'm not terribly interested in rational, outside reality. I was reading this book about constructivist architects, and it's so boring. I'm far more interested in – what do you call it – the psychotic-symbolistic reality inside. That's far more exciting. I have accepted these L S D experiences as more real.

'The drawback to these trips is the psychological needs – I need to be loved. I had this girl, it was someone to sleep with afterwards, someone to hold on to. You get frightened when you're not able to deal with things when you're away. I am confident now that I can deal with any situation, but these people who go doing murders on L S D are a bit worrying.' (Laughs.)

'But I've been there myself. I had this friend who wanted to murder me. I was quite looking forward to it. The scenes I get on are so fantastic – the treacheries and betrayals, I lose all my friends!

'Once I took L S D in the morning and walked about London – the fantastic thing that day was that I was a tourist – not the way I looked, but the way I walked, you know like tourists do. It was fantastic all these buildings.

'I got hung up before I started on L S D, over my sculpture – I got hung up over colouring it. I could only do feeble vague colours. Now it's so simple, I don't know what all the fuss was about. I just colour them as if they were living animals. It's so easy.' Here he produced a slightly flattened green polystyrene ball with half a dozen pin holes in it. 'This is a satellite. Isn't it fantastic? This girl of mine. Once when I was on a trip I saw her as Cathy MacGowan' (a popular teenage announcer on a defunct television show *Ready Steady Go*) 'with funny dried-up teeth. She did look so odd.

'The trouble with junkies is that it's all flashing and popping in their heads but they can't concentrate and get it out. It's terribly frustrating. I don't go much on drugs, I suppose because as an artist I want to be in control. There's another problem for junkies – all they think about is junk; they're not interested in people except as a means to getting junk. But they know so much about themselves – just for example, if you're trying to stop smoking, there are all these little scenes passing sweet shops and tobacconists and so on. Well, the junkie knows all this only a hundred times stronger.

'The first trip I was ever on – in Germany in this vast pine wood, I took a great lump of mescaline and walked by the lake until I felt its effects. You're frightened but you don't know how to be frightened – you can feel all the nerves, all down your finger nails and behind your teeth. You know, it's like your first bunk-up's terrifying, only this is much more so. Then I set off towards this tower on the hill – typical! – I don't realize it's bloody miles. Then it got dark – whoosh –' (he waves his hands downwards) '– I've never seen it get dark so fast. All the fairy stories, Cinderella and the big bad wolf in the pines. I was petrified, I've never been so frightened. But it was an I've been here before feeling, I suppose like nightmares. It was most peculiar, this feeling being too well known.

'As I say, I used to go on trips three times a week for a while; but now I've lost interest. I gave my last lot of LSD away to a bloke – I suppose because he'd never tried to hustle any off me.' He gave the impression of disconnected, slightly irritated concentration on his own internal processes that is typical of young artists or mild schizophrenics.

It is interesting that in this, the first period in which people have cut themselves off from religion and socially acceptable mystical experiences, drug-taking has become a major problem. For the first time in our history, there are no mechanisms for relating the supernatural, visions and ecstasies, to ordinary life. They are taken instead as symptoms of sickness. It seems likely that many young people use LSD, marihuana, amphetamines, according to their education, personality and opportunity, in attempts to fill the void twentieth-century living leaves inside the mind.

Illicit American use of hallucinogens is better documented. Use of hallucinogens in New York follows the lines of marihuana in being confined to more or less closed social groups; the activity associated with it seems to be more varied, perhaps because the drug is newer. At some LSD parties 'everyone is sitting about and waiting like on New Year's Eve, for something to happen.' At others there are solemn, silent basket makings and a religious atmosphere, at others again there are sexual orgies, 'if you fondle a woman's breast she becomes the whole breast ... the orgasm – it feels as though it's spilling right out of you.' The black market in the hallucinogens is rather loosely organized, with friends supplying each other and covering their costs, rather than an organized network of pushers. The non-addictiveness of the drugs makes for a fluctuation in demand that hardly attracts the established operators, who prefer the stability of the opiate market.

A particularly stupid use of LSD is to give it to an ignorant subject. The story of the girl at a party who had some put in her drink as an aphrodisiac, found animals crawling up her arms and jumped to her death out of a fourth floor window, is a hardy chestnut, although it may have some basis in fact. Certainly the drug has been used for seductions or simply as a joke. A newspaper story, in April 1966, described a group of people drinking in a pub who suddenly began hallucinating and behaving oddly. Another girl, going to Scotland to meet her future parents-in-law, was given a secret dose by a London 'practitioner' just before she set out, and had to endure a most alarming journey and a most difficult interview with these people who were to be rather important to her. The stress of the LSD experience and the risk of psychosis is obviously much higher when the subject has no idea what is happening. For what these are worth, the victim has considerable legal remedies: secret drug administration may be both a crime under the Offences against the Person Act* and a civil wrong for which a jury would certainly give very heavy damages. A practical joke which caused an incapacitating psychosis might cost the joker as much as a car accident – perhaps £30,000 – without the benefit of insurance.

In America, as one might expect, the illicit use of LSD has become almost institutionalized. There is a journal, sometimes of a high standard, called the *Psychedelic Review*.† There are a number of quasi-religious groups using the drugs; the best known is centred on Timothy Leary who, as this is written, has come into sharp conflict with the American Establishment over drug use, and was last reported advising his followers to renounce the hallucinogens. But the earlier history of his movement is interesting. Blum gives an account of some aspects in *Utopiates*.[2] (It must at once be said that the largest part of this book, devoted to the analysis of five groups of LSD users, is based on such tendentious material that very little reliance can be placed on it. The samples used are small, there is no guarantee of representativeness, and the subjects' reactions to the questionnaire seem coloured by the expectations of the interviewers.)

The most striking impression given by the descriptive parts of this book is that the LSD movement is much more a reaction

*This Act of 1861 provides that it is a felony, punishable with imprisonment for life, to administer, or attempt to administer, 'chloroform, laudanum, or other stupefying or overpowering drug matter or thing' in order to procure the commission of an indictable offence, e.g. rape. It further provides that it is a felony, punishable with up to ten years imprisonment, to administer unlawfully and maliciously 'any poison or other destructive or noxious thing' to anyone so as to endanger his life or to inflict upon him grievous bodily harm. The Sexual Offences Act 1966 adds another safeguard: 'It is an offence for a person to apply or administer to, or cause to be taken by, a woman any drug, matter or thing with intent to stupefy or overpower her so as thereby to enable any man to have unlawful sexual intercourse with her.'

†Available at a few London booksellers, or at $2 a copy, plus postage, from the publishers: Psychedelic Book Service, Box 171, New Hyde Park, New York, U.S.A.

against the American way of life – rather similar in some ways to the beatnik or folk-song cults – than a result of the pharmacology of the drug. It is observed that

> LSD is mainly used by professionals, intellectuals, or other middle-class people – in other words by people who are socially favoured, respected and generally conforming.... If LSD represents for them some kind of a revolt, it is a quiet one.... More and more people 'want out', and this includes, strikingly enough as the study shows, people who have been successful in society and have received the rewards that it promised them.

Some American LSD users take as a manual the *Tibetan Book of the Dead*,[18] annotated in *The Psychedelic Experience*.[19] This passage seems to explain the authors' intentions:

> Following the Tibetan model then, we distinguish three phases of the psychic experience. The first period, *Chikhai Bardo*, is that of complete transcendence – beyond words, beyond space-time, beyond self. There are no visions, no sense of self, no thoughts. There are only pure awareness and ecstatic freedom from all game (and biological) involvements.* The second lengthy period involves self, or external game reality, *Chönyld Bardo*, in sharp exquisite clarity or in the form of hallucinations (karmic apparitions). The final stage, *Sidpa Bardo*, involves the return to routine game reality and the self.
>
> For most persons the second (aesthetic or hallucinatory stage) is the longest. For the initiated the first stage of illumination lasts longer. For the unprepared, the heavy game players, those who anxiously cling to their egos, and for those who take the drug in a non-supportive setting, the struggle to regain reality begins early and usually lasts to the end of their session.... One purpose of this manual is to enable the person to regain the transcendence of First Bardo and to avoid prolonged entrapments in hallucinatory or ego-dominated game patterns.

On the cover of the book there is an explanation of how the authors, Leary and Alpert, were forced to leave Harvard. They comment, presumably with this and other episodes in mind:

---

*'"Games" are behavioural sequences defined by roles, rituals, goals, strategies, values, language, characteristic space-time locations and characteristic patterns of movement. Any behaviour not having these nine features is a non-game: this includes physiological reflexes, spontaneous play, and transcendent awareness.'[19]

... Westerners do not accept the existence of conscious processes for which they have no operational terms. The attitude which is prevalent is: if you can't label it, and if it is beyond current notions of space-time and personality, then it is not open for investigation. Thus we see the ego-loss experience confused with schizophrenia. Thus we see present-day psychiatrists solemnly pronouncing the psychedelic keys as psychosis-producing and dangerous.[19]

Devotees of this and other cults have been criticized elsewhere:

Among the effects of the drug are (1) disassociation and detachment ('initiates begin to show a certain blandness or superiority, or feeling of being above and beyond the normal world of social reality'), (2) interpersonal insensitivity ('inability to predict in advance what the social reaction to a "psilocybin party" would be'), (3) omniscience, religious and philosophical naïveté ('many reports are given of deep mystical experiences but their chief characteristic is the wonder at one's own profundity rather than a genuine concern to probe deeper into the experience of the human race in these matters'), (4) impulsivity ('one of the most difficult parts of the research has been to introduce any order into who takes psilocybin under what conditions. Any controls have either been rejected as interfering with the warmth necessary to have a valuable experience, or accepted as desirable but then not applied because somehow an occasion arises when it seems "right" to have a psilocybin session').[20]

Whether the use of hallucinogens will develop along these lines in Britain is impossible to say. In the two years since this chapter was written, the frenzied first interest in L S D and psychedelics has died down, probably because once a person has taken half a dozen trips, he has had all the drug has to offer. Moreover, since each experience takes twelve hours, and the after effects are felt for days, it's a very time-consuming operation. The professional people likely to be interested in the drug are unable to afford the amount of time needed. Continued and widespread use of the drug is something we are likely to have to take into account, and it will be necessary to devise intelligent policies towards it.

10
Identification, Cure and the End of Addiction

In the first edition of this book there was nothing about identifying addicts, because at the time this was not seen as a problem. By a kind of social tautology, the only 'addicts' in existence were the ones one knew about, and they, by definition, were the patients of doctors. Although everyone said that the Home Office figures for addicts, totalled from reports by medical, police, prison and probation services, were underestimates, no one had undertaken the detective work necessary to uncover the secret users.

That was true until the publication of Rathod and de Alarcón's excellent investigations[19, 20] into the addict population of Crawley (see p. 36 above). They, psychiatrists working in the local psychiatric service, suspected, quite rightly, that the eight known addicts in Crawley didn't represent the entire population. They developed and tested five ways of compiling a true list. These were: 1. The probation service, whose officers were asked to pass on the names and addresses of anyone known to be using drugs. 2. The police, who passed on the names of people convicted of possessing heroin, the names of those searched in the street on suspicion of possessing heroin, and the names of those associating with known drug users. 3. Known heroin users who were patients of the writers were encouraged to tell them about other users. 4. A survey was made of all hospitals and general practices in the area for patients between fifteen and twenty-five who had had jaundice (a frequent result of unsterile injections) within the last two years. 5. On the assumption that heroin users are likely to be pan-addicts and not necessarily too careful what they take, a search of all hospital casualty department records for people in this age group admitted with overdoses of hypnotics or stimulants.

This was in addition to the 'normal' detection methods of drug addicts presenting to their G.P.s and court referrals for psychiatric reports.

All this information was collated onto one card for each subject. A typical card would run: 'Jaundice, 12 December 1966; named by heroin user 5 May 1967; named by second heroin user 15 June 1967; police suspect 23 September 1967; G.P. referral 5 October 1967; seen in outpatients' clinic 8 October 1967.'

Interestingly, they found that the two most productive screening methods were information from other heroin users, which produced first evidence on 46 people, and the jaundice survey, first evidence on 20. G.P. referrals produced first evidence on only 8 of 92 users. The casualty survey produced 15, police suspicions 3, convictions 4, and the probation service 2.

The same writers followed up this work with a study of clinical signs of heroin dependence, which included a useful investigation into the 'oddities of behaviour and appearance which [a group of twenty parents] had noticed in their children before the use of drugs came to light'. These parents had noticed the following signs (the percentages refer to the number of parents reporting each sign):

Poor appetite: 80%
No interest in personal appearance: 70%
Unexpected absences from home (to obtain supply): 65%
Spends long periods in his room: 65%
Sleeps out (loses motivation to come home when high): 65%
Slow and halting speech: 60%
Gives up organized activities: 60%
Receives and makes frequent phone calls (to check on supplies): 55%
Blood spotting on clothes (mainly pyjama tops and shirts): 50%
Litter in room or pockets: 45%
Stooped posture: 45%
Fully burnt matches lying around (e.g. floating in toilet) used to prepare the fix: 20%
Teaspoons lying around (used to prepare fix): 15%

'When the parents found out about their child's predicament

and began to attend our groups, many of them became aware of changes in general behaviour – e.g. one parent told us, "In the last two days his usual breakfast appetite has gone, he must be taking drugs again"; another said "The frequent telephone calls have started again". In both cases their suspicions were later confirmed.'

This paper goes on to distinguish the symptoms of addiction from those of other adolescent problems. Incipient schizophrenia produces many of the symptoms noted above, but doesn't lead to making new friends; depressions too, but again sufferers are unlikely to be dreamy, euphoric or spend nights out. Disappointing love affairs produce irritability and preoccupation. 'All these possibilities have to be kept in mind when considering dependence on drugs, otherwise parents may be alarmed unnecessarily. On the other hand, if many of these signs occur together, and there have been recent changes in general behaviour, drug dependence should be high on the list of differential diagnosis.'

Cure

The 'cure' of addiction presents two problems, one physical, and the other social and psychological. The first arises only with the truly addictive drugs – opiates and barbiturates – which produce physical changes and dependence in the body. Although a great deal is said about this physical aspect of drug cures, it is in fact a relatively minor matter. Taking heroin and the opiates first, the problem of reducing an addict's dosage to zero can be solved in several ways. One is simply to cut off his supplies, to let him go 'cold-turkey', and fight his way through the withdrawal as best he can. Though quick, and offering the advantage that he is too weak to run away until fairly over his physical dependence, this method is now considered too brutal for use in medical practice. Régimes for gradual withdrawal vary according to the institution and the doctor administering them. They divide again into those that employ a substitute drug, and those that do not. Much fuss is made over 'heroin cures', meaning drugs that can be substituted for heroin without producing further addiction – as heroin was at first substituted for morphine – but it does not seem that they are anything more than a convenience, and whether they are used or not has no real bearing on the final outcome. In the American Public Health Hospitals at Fort Worth and Lexington, methadone – a synthetic and less active opiate – is given by mouth in decreasing doses; in other systems the actual drug of addiction is progressively reduced in quantity. At the same time vitamins and tranquillizers may be given, and sleeping pills at night, which may have to be continued for some months to combat the ex-addict's insomnia. In any event there is no need for the addict to feel more than the discomfort of a sharp dose of flu during a modern medically supervised withdrawal. In H.M. prisons the treatment followed is left to the discretion of the medical officer, but it is usual to withdraw drugs according to the general principles outlined above.[1]

Any addict who will stay, or can be kept, under supervision and without being able to get at drugs for ten days can be restored to a normal metabolic state. It may take another three months of rest, good food and exercise to put him back in reasonable physical condition. Medical science has gone this far; it has not begun to attack the problem of drug dependence.

As we have seen in earlier chapters, the person who is dependent on drugs – whether they are addictive or not – is the end result of many years of damaging pressures. He probably comes from a bad, cold home, he has no self-confidence, no belief in his own identity, no experience of normal living and normal satisfactions, and, on the contrary, powerful impressions of the pleasures to be got from drugs. The very first problem after withdrawal is that he has nothing to do all day, and no one to talk to.

As a habit takes hold, other interests lose importance to the user. Life telescopes down to junk, one fix and looking forward to the next, 'stashes' and 'scripts', 'spikes' and 'droppers'. The addict himself often feels that he is leading a normal life and that junk is incidental. He does not realize that he is just going through the motions in his non-junk activities.[2]

And again:

... it's like telling a man afflicted with infantile paralysis to run a hundred yards. Without the stuff Tom's face takes on a strained expression; as the effects of the last fix wear off all grace dies within him. He becomes a dead thing. For him, ordinary consciousness is like a slow desert at the centre of his being; his emptiness is suffocating. He tries to drink, to think of women, to remain interested, but his expression becomes shifty. The one vital coil in him is the bitter knowledge that he can choose to fix again. I have watched him. At the beginning he is over-confident. He laughs too much. But soon he falls silent and hovers restlessly at the edge of a conversation, as though he were waiting for the void of the drugless present to be miraculously filled. (*What would you do all day if you didn't have to look for a fix?*) He is like a child dying of boredom, waiting for promised relief, until his expression becomes sullen. Then when his face takes on a distasteful expression, I know he has decided to go and look for a fix.[3]

Whether he remains off drugs after withdrawal depends crucially on his morale and motivation, and these depend entirely on his relationship with his doctor. The successful addict curer has to combine the qualities of gaoler and wild-animal catcher, to be gentle yet more single-minded than the monomaniacs he has to deal with. One of the dozen London doctors who dealt with addicts before Treatment Centres started reports that she follows an elaborate preparatory routine before embarking on dose reduction. The addict is at first given unlimited drugs to establish confidence and binding ties. Then he is made to conform to a set dose, then to a reduced dose. At the same time he is helped and encouraged, even being lent money if necessary, to get a home, find a job, settle down, keep away from other addicts, and generally to begin learning what ordinary life is about. Psychiatric treatment begins:

The goal ... is to correct as far as possible these personality difficulties, to give the patient a sense of security, self-reliance and self-confidence and a sense of responsibility towards himself, his family and friends, and towards the community, and to replace his sense of anxiety and insecurity with a sense of well-being. ... At the same time it was made clear that insight was not enough; that a constructive attempt must be made to control and strengthen the weaknesses of a personality which had been led to disaster. Even those few young patients who had been led into taking drugs out of curiosity and through the influence of bad companions were made to realize that the danger was due to a personality disorder which must be rectified.[4]

Three hospitals in and around London accept addicts for treatment, but there seem to be few attempts made at adequate preparation before withdrawal, or even more important, at the intensive social support needed after withdrawal. The success rates are in line with those reported from institutions in America and other parts of the world: 16 per cent free for seven years according to one writer,[5] or 10 per cent.[6] The importance of strong character and motivation in the therapist is shown by the relatively higher success rates claimed by Anglican nuns who run a nursing home at Spelthorne St Mary's (near Egham in Surrey). This establishment accepts female addicts and alcoholics, who are encouraged to stay for some months in the community for rehabilitation after withdrawal. Because of their vocations and personal stability the nuns seem able to give considerable emotional support to their patients, and ex-patients often form very strong attachments to the place. At every weekend it is common to find one or two there on a visit, and at Christmas there are likely to be more visitors than patients. Apart from the hospitals that offer out-patient treatment centres and the three or so that accept addicts as in-patients, there is a number of half-way houses, day centres, and other more or less loose organizations designed to help and support addicts. These wax and wane with the enthusiasms of their promoters, but cannot be said to offer together more than a palliative to the basic problems of drug dependence.

The comparative rarity of British addicts in the past has meant that there was neither need nor material for the elaborate comparative studies of cure methods and successes that are necessary before any realistic policy towards addiction can be devised. As usual, we have to turn to the superior resources of the United States.

Since the typical American addict is now a twenty-year-old Negro boy living in a big city[7] their experience can be suggestive only. It has been mentioned that the cure and study of addiction is regarded as a Federal responsibility. The two public-health hospitals (see p. 31) are open to voluntary and prison patients. An attempt is made to rehabilitate both classes by work in the hospital; voluntary patients are expected to stay for a minimum of five months at Lexington. About one patient in six is a prisoner. A follow-up over twelve years of a hundred addicts discharged from treatment at Lexington in 1952–3 shows several interesting facts about the relative effectiveness of different régimes. Of this hundred, many were in Lexington more than once either as voluntary patients or prisoners in the years after 1953. There were altogether 270 voluntary admissions, but only eleven times did these patients stay off drugs for more than a year after treatment. Almost as many did as well themselves, going cold-turkey at home. The most effective treatment turned out to be a prison sentence of more than eight months followed by more than a year's parole – but the prison sentence without parole was hardly more effective than voluntary treatment:

... the likelihood that significant abstinence would occur after prolonged involuntary imprisonment followed by prolonged involuntary supervision was *fifteen* times greater than after voluntary hospitalization.

And long hospitalization, produced most often by court pressure, produced longer abstinence than short hospitalization.

The importance of coercion in treating addicts seems widely underestimated. The author of this paper says:

The findings of this paper suggest that addicts may differ from most psychiatric patients. ... In general psychiatric patients cannot be ordered to give up symptoms, and prolonged hospitalization drives patients towards increased dependence rather than maturity. ...

Addicts tolerate anxiety poorly; they 'act out'; they often engage in self-destructive behaviour that is not consciously realized as detrimental. Individuals with such defences often do not experience a strong conscious desire to change. ...

Psychotherapy is most often directed towards relieving or correcting unrewarding behaviour that has arisen out of too much, or the wrong sort of training. The delinquent addict, however, has often encountered *too little* consistent concern from authority rather than too much or the wrong sort. The professional permissiveness of the psychiatrist may seem to threaten the addict's immature efforts to control his impulses. Both at Lexington and at the Riverside Hospital in New York, patients not uncommonly ask for more controls, not fewer. A 1the same time there is little to suggest that punishment *per se* either deters or benefits the addict . . .* He needs someone to *care* when he is honest and independent.[8]†

Addicts are notoriously resistant to ordinary psychotherapy. One way of looking at this is to observe that analysis depends on communication, on the patient's acceptance of the therapist as a real human being who can have a real effect on him. But the addict's whole life is organized to remove any dependence on humanity; given his drugs, he is self-sufficient, able to generate his own satisfactions and guilts and to live a rich emotional life independent of the outside world. He therefore has no motives for communication when things are going well; when he does present himself for treatment it is often not because he wants to be cured of addiction, but because his addiction is not working as it should.‡ He is a two-time loser who wants to get back to being a one-time loser; not to take the much more perilous step to being an unloser. The ordinary psychiatric patient is like a burr, offering many hooks to the world and the therapist – often too many; the therapist's best strategy is to stand still and let his patient attach himself as he will. But the addict is like a nut; smooth with a thick armour. The only hook he offers is his need for drugs, and that can be satisfied in a number of ways. To reach the addict, his shell must be cracked. We might guess that it would be necessary to counter the coercion of opiates with the coercion of therapy; it is noticeable that those London doctors who treat addicts often have strong, obdurate personalities,[9] in contrast to the majority of psychiatrists, and that their writings

---

*The success of prolonged imprisonment in treating the addicts reported was due simply to keeping them in contact with therapy.

†During my interview with the author of the paper quoted on p. 139 n.4 an ex-addict who had been out of treatment for some years rang to tell her he was a father. His son was barely an hour old. 'There,' she said, 'that's the sort of relationship you've got to have to help addicts.'

‡I owe this idea to Dr Salomon Resnik.

often show authoritarian tones – for example the writer quoted above and on p. 143.

Another successful American treatment centre, Synanon, an informal self-help community of addicts and ex-addicts, also seems to rely on force for its operation. The organization was founded in 1958 by an ex-alcoholic member of Alcoholics Anonymous. In 1966 it had 450 members. An addict who wishes to join first has to withdraw cold-turkey as an earnest of his good faith. He is then required to live in the community for a minimum of two years. The central features of the treatment are the seminars – mispronounced 'synanons' by an early illiterate member – where the members meet in groups of eight or twelve for one and a half hours three times a week and subject each other to the most searching and vicious criticism, abuse and ridicule. The members of each seminar are rotated so that all the community come under fire from one another. Since it is one of the most characteristic personality problems of addicts that they cannot bear disparagement, this daily discovery that one can be criticized and still live on amicable terms with one's attackers must be a most salutary lesson. As well as this cathartic 'gut' experience, the members have a positive frame of society to live in that also deeply understands their problems. They work, and are paid a small amount of pocket money. They have the prospect of rising to the Board of Management. People who seem not to be benefiting from the community are given the choice of expulsion or trial by their peers. If they choose trial and are found guilty the men have their heads shaved; women have to wear a placard round their necks: 'I am a returnee from the twilight zone.' Desperate appliances relieve desperate diseases; Synanon has the motto 'Hang Tough' and claims a success rate of fifty per cent.[10]

Daytop (Drug Addicts Treated On Probation) Village is an offspring of Synanon, with much the same organization. In 1967 it had a membership of ninety people, all ex-addicts. It understands the problems of the addicts' personality and takes a strong line with them. Barry Sugarman, describing Daytop in *New Society*,[21] writes:

In very forceful terms the entering addict is told by senior members of Daytop that he is responsible for what he has done and that he cannot slough it off on unloving parents, negligent teachers, a corrupt society or any of the usual culprits. He decided to take dope and to steal and lie to get the money for it. He is also told that the reason he is an addict is because he is a child in terms of character and emotional development. Therefore they will treat him like a child at first: he must obey all the many rules of the house and all the decisions of the senior members without question. He may not leave the house, write letters, make phone calls, have visitors: he must perform the tasks assigned to him which at first will be the most menial household cleaning chores: cooking pots, floors, lavatories.

Another variant of the basic Synanon idea, but apparently more democratic in its organization, is found in the Phoenix Houses of New York. They claim a success rate of 80 per cent, and one opened in London under the wing of the Maudsley Hospital in 1970.

A fourth regime, which also uses cured addicts, backed by the sanctions of the courts, to wrestle with the uncured is New York State's programme under which addicts convicted of any crime can be committed to a clinic for up to five years. The system was developed in Puerto Rico by Dr Efran Ramirez.

In the light of these views, the Brain Committee's second report reads curiously:

Para. 24 . . . we are mindful of the obstinacy of some addicts and the likelihood that some of them will not attend a treatment centre. Since *compulsory treatment meets with little success* [author's italics] there is little that can be done for these people beyond restricting the possibility of illicit supplies. Others may want to break off treatment after they have embarked on it. This may be a short-lived feature caused by the discomfort of the withdrawal symptoms. We think that the staff of a treatment centre should have powers to enable them compulsorily to detain such a patient during such a crisis. This we appreciate would require legislation.[11]

To withdraw an addict, even forcibly, but then to leave him virtually on his own, is as useful as pulling a broken leg straight, and then expecting its owner to walk away. The Brain Committee realized that 'the situation would in our view be greatly improved if there were proper facilities for long-term rehabilitation, both psychological and physical, in the treatment centres and elsewhere. To go into more detail about this would be outside our term of reference . . .' (para. 25). All the material discussed above suggests that something much more drastic is needed; how this is to be achieved without alienating addicts and creating an even more virulent sub-culture is discussed in the next chapter.

An interesting new approach to the cure of heroin addicts is simply to transfer them to another, slower acting drug. No attempt is made to wean them from drugs altogether, but because the substitute drug that is often used, methadone, has a span of 24–35 hours as against heroin's 8 hours, their lives are transformed. Instead of being constantly busy (see p. 46) they now have time to work, eat and live something of a family life. Also because tolerance to methadone produces cross tolerance to heroin the ex-addict can get no 'high' however much heroin he takes. He gets his substitute from a clinic, and so it is possible to break his contacts with the drug sub-culture. Dole and Nyswander in New York have 800 addicts, all with four years' or more experience of main-lining and several attempts at cures, on this regime. The treatment begins with six weeks in hospital getting rested up, assessed and transferred to methadone. The patients are given the largest daily dose that doesn't make them sleepy – this prevents escalation onto heroin. After this they live out, helped by massive psychiatric and social care, go to a clinic every day for their dose of methadone and leave a urine sample as a check against other drug use. This lasts a year. In the third phase, when they have settled down as functioning members of society, they go once a week to get their doses. It is accepted that they will probably never be able to do without drugs, but in this they are like diabetics. It doesn't much matter.

Acupuncture, which is said to cure almost any disease, is also reported to be effective against heroin addiction. A treatment centre in Kowloon claims to have cured 600 addicts by passing a 125Hz, 5V electric wave through the conchae of their ears.[23] (I tried it, without perceiving any effect, but then, I am not an addict.) An English doctor involved in the experiments plans to

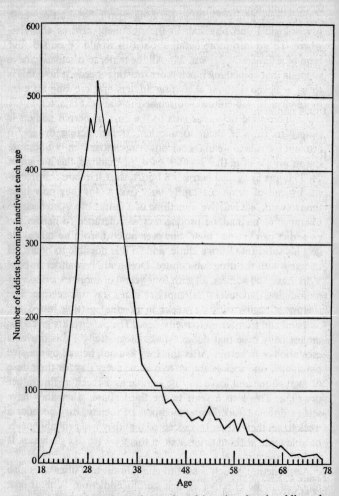

Figure 3. This curve shows the *number* of American heroin addicts who appear to give up using drugs, plotted against their *age*. Since addiction seldom starts before sixteen, this graph shows that the vast majority give up their habit in the first ten years.

set up a unit here to continue the work.[24] But before one concludes that the addiction problem is solved, it might be as well to remember that, as for U.S. conscripts in Vietnam (p. 34), life for the average Chinese in overcrowded Hong Kong is so tiresome that, even in the absence of fundamental psychic predisposition, heroin addiction may be an attractive strategy for dealing with it. British addicts probably need the drug much more and are that much harder to cure.

So far this chapter has dealt with opiate addiction. Much the same techniques are used in withdrawing barbiturates, except that, because of the risk of convulsions and possible death, the daily reduction must be made smaller and the period of reduction extended to three weeks or more. The patient should never be allowed to walk about unattended, and the doctor should be

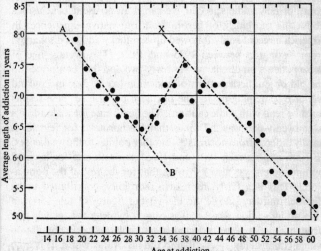

Figure 4. Here the average *duration* of addiction is plotted against the *age* at which addicts started using drugs. Two different types of addiction seem to be defined by the lines AB and XY. On each of these, the later one starts, the less time one serves as an addict. This evidence suggests that addicts mature out of drug use in some way or other. Both curves after Winick.[16]

constantly ready to give a holding dose to prevent withdrawal.[12] The subsequent problems are presumably the same.

Untreated Addiction

If an addict is not cured – and few are – one can say with some certainty that sooner or later he will either give up drugs or die. But the morbidity of drugs is uncertain; numbers are too few to calculate death and suicide rates accurately, even if the population at risk were known.

A survey by Bewley of the 507 heroin addicts known to the Home Office between 1954 and 1964 shows, in spite of the fact that there were seven times as many at the end of the decade as there had been at the beginning, a curiously constant rate of death at about two a year.[13] This is probably explained by the youth of new addicts; so far we can draw no useful conclusions about the morbidity of heroin from our native experience. In America a recent study followed up Kentucky addicts discharged from Lexington between 1935 and 1959. (The average age of these patients on discharge was forty-two and they conformed to the old or southern pattern of addiction (see p. 31); in England we have something nearer the northern pattern, so these results must be read with some caution). The death-rate for male addicts over twenty-five was 2.7 times that for normals; for females it hardly differed from normals[14] – another pointer to the weaker sex. In Formosa between 1901 and 1935 the death-rate for licensed opium addicts was also 2·7 times that for the rest of the population.[15] This is a fairly impressive morbidity, contributed to by disease, murder, suicide, accidents; but figures of this sort can give no indication whether it is caused by drug use, or whether drug use, as it were, selected a particularly weak population which is unusually susceptible to the ills of this world. It is even conceivable that addicts might die quicker if they were not calmed and immobilized for a large part of their lives. In fact this may positively contribute to addicts' longevity. A recent government study in America showed that although heroin addicts drove nearly twice as many miles a year as the ordinary American

(18,000 miles as against 10,000), mostly in order to get their drugs, they had half as many car accidents, even though they would almost all make the return journey in a state of euphoria. The moral is that calm saves lives on the road, even if it is pharmacological.

It is commonly thought that addiction to heroin ends inevitably in the addict's dissolution and death. It is not impossible that this is folk-lore rather than fact. The evolution of the addict's relationship with opiates, and its possibilities as a self-limiting process, are explored in two important papers by Winick. He concludes intriguingly that for two thirds of addicts the use of opiates is a process that lasts for a comparatively short part of their lives. He finds, on examining the records held by the Federal Bureau of Narcotics of 7,234 addicts who had been active in 1955 and had not been reported by 1960, that the average length of addiction is 8·6 years. Analysis showed that addiction lasted on the average from the early twenties to about thirty-five. The graph reproduced here, Figure 3, shows that a large number of addicts drop out after a very short period of use. An even more interesting curve, Figure 4, shows the relationship between the length of addiction and the age at which addiction begins. Cases whose addiction lasted more than sixteen years have been omitted; but for the majority of addicts it appears that the duration of drug use is very simply related to the age of starting. The earlier you start, the longer you go on. It also suggests that there are two great groups of addicts: the 'adolescent' and the 'middle-aged' – perhaps corresponding to the northern and southern patterns of addiction. The decrease in duration of addiction with later starting is extremely consistent, with a correlation of $-\cdot95$ on the adolescent line, and $-\cdot80$ on the other. The points in between turn out to be averages between the two. The curves are so regular that Winick deduces simple formulae to predict the probable length of an individual's addiction:

If L = length of addiction and a = age
for those aged between 19 and 35
$$L = 10 \cdot 09 - 0 \cdot 126a$$

153

$$\text{for those aged between 38 and 60}$$
$$L = 11 \cdot 58 - 0 \cdot 107a$$

One hopes that such regularity shows more than happy mathematical neatness, and proclaims a buried natural law. Winick supposes that this dropping out is the result of a process of maturing; that the earlier in each group an addict begins drug use, the more intense his problems are and the longer it takes him to grow out of them. The two ages from which the longest periods of addiction are likely are 18 and 37, both ages of greater stress for American men. He points out that at 18 the adolescent is confronted with the problems of deciding what sort of person he is; at 37 the man is faced with accepting what he has become. At the one age decisions *must* be made; at the other they have become irrelevant. He also points out that the curve in Figure 3 is identical in shape and distribution to the drop-out curve for psychotics, and very similar to that for recidivism among juvenile delinquents. It is possible that drugs, delinquency, psychosis are different methods of dealing with the same problems.[16] But before we follow this line of thought, it is necessary to consider some criticism of Winick's work. There are two major assumptions: first, that an addict inevitably appears in the Bureau's file, as it claims, within five years of beginning drug use – there is no independent evidence in support of this; second, that non-appearance in the file means non-addiction.

At first glance, one might suppose that the high death-rates reported by O'Donnell and Tu would imply that all the drop-outs were in fact dead. But if one works backwards from Winick's survivors, using a death-rate 2·7 times the normal, one finds that his 4,000-odd addicts would, on this assumption, be the remnants of more initial users than the entire population of the U.S.A.

A follow-up of Puerto Rican opiate addicts in New York designed to test the maturation theory found that two thirds were still addicted, and that their drug use had tended to increase over the years. But on the other hand the rest had become abstinent, had given up their criminal behaviour and had become reasonably productive citizens. About half were steadily employed and

90 per cent had not been arrested in the previous three years. The authors of this paper conclude:

It appears, then, that two major patterns exist with respect to the life course of opiate addiction in the United States. In one instance the addict becomes increasingly enmeshed in a non-productive or criminal career as his dependence on opiates increases into adult years. In the second case, the addict terminates his drug-centred way of life and assumes, or re-establishes, a legitimate role in society. In this latter sense, it may be said that some one third of opiate addicts mature out of their dependence on drugs.[22]

If, after a certain period of addiction, the criminal and 'straight' ways of life compete for addicts, that would be another excellent reason why we should try to avoid driving drug use any further underground.

It must of course be remembered in attempting to apply these results to our experience, that few American addicts actually have access to any quantity of opiates, and that few in consequence have well-developed physical habits. It would perhaps be more accurate to say that most American addicts are no more than drug dependent. On the other hand English addicts, supplied with pure heroin, are able to build up really massive habits, and have their freedom of action very much reduced (see p. 173 below). But it is not uncommon for users of up to a grain a day in England to give their habit up. In the course of my own casual inquiries I was told of nine who had done so.

There is obviously not enough evidence to say with any certainty whether addicts use opiates for a while, and give them up when their emotional needs have passed; or whether they are grabbed and held, unwilling, by the drug. More research is essential; here we can only speculate on the consequences of Winick's interpretation.

One wonders, then, whether it is any use trying to 'cure' addicts simply by withdrawal, before they are ripe to give up drugs. It is possible that the normal 10 per cent cure rate for this method is due simply to people who would have ended their addiction anyway. It may even be harmful in certain cases to prevent the addict using heroin. We are so accustomed to consider drugs as unmitigated evils that it is worth rehearsing the argument leading to this conclusion.

1. Some pre-addicts (see p. 48) sound very like some young pre-schizophrenics described by Laing. Both groups were 'good' – i.e. passive – babies, often coming from homes that were materially not too badly off, both had strong but ambivalent relationships with their mothers, but ineffective fathers, both showed extremely plastic personalities.

2. Laing suggests that schizophrenia is the rest of a long attempt to evade deep anxiety, guilt and insecurity caused by the individual's failure to conceive of himself as a real, solid human being. He builds a false and variable personality front; he pretends to behave as people seem to want him to. Eventually the vacuum inside this shield becomes so large that the individual is cut off from reality and becomes mad.[17]

3. Heroin (see p. 21) is a specific against anxiety and painful emotions.

4. It is possible that the sort of person who uses heroin to obliterate his worries might otherwise embark on the schizophrenic's manoeuvres to avoid them.

5. Winick's work suggests that the heroin addict is likely to mature out of addiction as his instinctual drives die down, as the social pressures on him lessen, and perhaps – since he is relieved of tension by the drug – as he completes the learning processes he could not in childhood.

6. The schizophrenic, once his disease has been acute for more than a year, is likely to suffer irreversible damage, and is – in the present state of psychiatry – incurable.

7. Perhaps it is better that he should be a drug addict for nine years or so, with at least the chance of some social function during this time, and a two to three chance of eventual recovery, than to be mad for a lifetime.

8. It may be possible that premature withdrawal from drugs re-exposes the addict to schizophrenia.

Laing writes, in a letter to the author,

From my own clinical practice, I have had the impression on a number of occasions that the use of heroin might be forestalling a schizophrenic-like psychosis. For some people heroin seems to enable them to step from the whirling periphery of the gyroscope, as it were, nearer to the still centre within themselves;

and he suggests the usefulness of surveys to discover if the use of heroin were less among schizophrenics than among the population at large, and if the incidence of schizophrenia were less among addicts.

In the present state of public opinion it would require some hardihood in a psychiatrist to addict his adolescent schizophrenic patients. The nearest reference in the literature seems to be the already quoted account of opium use to pacify violent insane criminals in nineteenth-century America.[18] Opium is also said to be given to delinquent children in Formosa, who subsequently grow out of both habits.

11
Control of Drugs

The control of illicitly used drugs poses a multitude of intractable problems. We do not know precisely their effect or their mode of action in the body; we cannot do more than guess about the strength, nature, purpose of the motives that cause some people to become dependent on drugs; we have even less idea of the probable effect of widespread drug use on our society. Here, as menacingly as anywhere in the field of public policy, the penalties for wrong decisions loom. Should one be liberal or penal? If neither, where in between? One can make out a case for the possibility of total social degeneracy and breakdown consequent on movement in either direction.

In particular, we fear to make the experiment of liberality; but whether we like it or not, the experiment is being made for us. Drugs are becoming part of the lives of people in every part of society: housewives in the Welsh valleys, school-children in Sheffield, artists in Cornwall, West Indians at High Wycombe, racing cyclists at Brentford, psychiatrists and their patients at Hendon; to all of these, drugs that were unknown to ordinary people in Britain a generation ago are becoming accepted accessories of life. Technological advance reaches inwards, and it is impossible to keep it in the hands of the Establishment. Regulations and attitudes towards drugs, formed when their illicit use was confined to a small, tractable minority, are now being strained. The purpose of this chapter, and indeed of this book, is not to advocate immediate, drastic changes to these social adaptations, but more to suggest new facts and attitudes for discussion: to help to make it possible to reorientate ourselves to considerable and increasing drug use.

The first problem is: *Why* do we want to control drugs? This is a hard question. Now that freer sexual behaviour is becoming assimilated into our moral system, it seems that drug-taking

158

is moving into its place as one of those matters that are defended or attacked with more than rational heat, a question to which considerations of logic are only marginally relevant. It is probably more useful, therefore, first to examine unconscious reasons for restricting drug use. These are various. An obvious motive is that someone under the influence of drugs can be frightening or angering; he is hard to recognize, and consequently his behaviour is unpredictable. It is not until one thinks of alcohol as a drug that one realizes how subtly we have adapted to its use. The drunk is immediately recognizable by the way he stands, by the expression of his face, by his gait, by the situation in which we find him, by the way he talks, even by his smell. We know very well how he is likely to behave, and we make great allowances for actions that would otherwise be unacceptable. There are other adaptations to alcohol: it is distinctively flavoured, so one could hardly take it in ignorance. It is diluted so that the process of getting it into the bloodstream takes time and some physical effort. It is expensive enough not to be used absolutely casually.

Drugs on the other hand are subject to few of these controls. Their users show no signs that are intelligible to the ordinary person. Because we do not understand the cues, we can only recognize users by their overtly anti-social acts. As a result the drug gets the blame that we would, in the case of alcohol, attach to the user. Here for example is a trivial news story:

DRUG TAKERS OVERTURN GRAVESTONES
Two young men who had taken drugs ran riot in Brookwood Cemetery, Surrey, late one night. . . . They pushed over forty-eight memorials with considerable force between 11 p.m. and 11.30 p.m. . . . causing damage estimated at £2,500. . . . On each of two charges of possessing a quantity of a drug (Cannabis Resin) without authority, they were given a conditional discharge.[1]

The ordinary reader must feel that something shocking has happened; he may be less sure where to put the blame. If the boys had been drunk, the situation is clear: they were wrong to get drunk, more wrong than to behave badly. But drugs – one is not certain. This doubt and ambivalence towards drugs – or more accurately, towards acts done under the influence of drugs, the only evidence people have of their existence – encourages drug users to assert their moral exemption, to claim that it was the drug that did the deed, not they. This in turn intensifies the alienation towards drugs, and makes it more difficult to develop the social adaptations to them that we have towards alcohol.

Such rejection of the possibility of human control over drugs in turn enables society to see the drug user as incurably different, and therefore as a scapegoat. This is stronger in America than here; but it is necessary to point it out as one of the consequences of penal control of drugs. Trocchi puts it well:

> It's a nice tangible cause for juvenile delinquency. And it lets most people out because they're alcoholics. There's an available pool of wasted-looking bastards to stand trial as corrupters of their children. It provides the police with something to do, and as junkies and pot-heads are relatively easy to apprehend because they have to take so many chances to get hold of their drugs, a heroic police can make spectacular arrests, lawyers can do a brisk business, judges can make speeches, the big peddlars can make fortunes, the tabloids can sell millions of copies. John Citizen can sit back and watch evil get its just deserts.[2]

Then, as we have seen, drug use is not simply a pharmacological affair between the user's body chemistry and an alien substance; it is the cause and effect of a sub-group of society, and in many cases the drug itself – or its visible accessories – are a part of social display. Young people in particular use drugs to demonstrate their rebellion and emancipation from their elders. However unconscious the message, society receives it loud and insulting. A passage in the *Utopiates*, describing American beatnik marihuana users who react against middle-class backgrounds by their dramatically squalid way of life, analyses one facet of society's reaction.

> We suggest that the police officer – or citizen – is, in fact, threatened by his quite accurate but partially unconscious understanding of what some users do mean or intend by their drug use. That threat mobilizes the individual's feelings about past trauma of his own, trauma experienced at the hands of parental authorities during the difficult stages

of learning order and suppressing impulse. These individuals respond with disgust, anger, revulsion and fear and 'cleanse' themselves by the standard human ploy of making the enemy external, that is of scape-goating. . . . The emotionally aroused police officer who calls these users 'dirty' and hates them for their 'self-indulgence' is quite an accurate diagnostician, even though the diagnosis is in the service of his own defence system.[3]

The problem of the rebellious, dependent young has always been to find something they can do without hurting themselves, that will still look dangerous enough to force their elders to stand and fight. For the moment drugs, particularly the soft drugs – marihuana, amphetamines – do the trick nicely.

So, another motive for society's interest in drug control is that here one finds something intimately connected with juvenile revolt that can be weighed, counted, analysed, held in the hand and sworn to in court. Something rather more satisfactory as evidence of young ingratitude than long hair and contemptuous expressions.

And finally, drugs that are thought to provide ecstasy, visions or even happiness and contentment without reference to one's material or social position, pose an obvious social threat. The cohesion of society and its control over its members depend on the inability of anyone to obtain satisfactions unless he pays for them: to pay for them he must earn, and in earning he conforms to the major rules of society. The trouble with the drug user is that he has found a way to escape from society's controls: he has no family to earn and care for, he has no self-respect, he has no home, he needs no job. Quite obviously, if more than a small minority of people lived as he does, our social system, held to-gether by the iron chains of mutual production and consumption, would fall apart. The results would be unpleasant for those who were not drug users, and so it is not surprising that those whose job it is to enforce the written and unwritten laws take a very dim view of illicit drug use. Heroin, the banisher of anxiety, is par-ticularly dangerous, since worry – over one's status, security, old age – is the mainspring of free enterprise capitalism. One works *oneself*, because one is dedicated and finds fulfilment in the service of society: one is not so sure about all the others. It is probably not a bad thing that they are spurred on by their anxiety over rent and retirement, the need to buy food and status-giving consumer durables. If anyone, after an injection or a pill costing a few pennies, were able to sit back and let the world go hang, where would we all be? On the other hand, equally dangerous drugs that support the social system by stupefying those who, like many housewives, would otherwise find it intolerable, are not seen to present any problem.

Paradoxically, the conscious grounds for drug control are far less easy to set out. We just do not know enough to separate the effects of drug use from the social conditions in which it is attractive. Thus, we can hardly use Hong Kong with its 300,000 addicts in a population of 4 millions as a model for British society if, for some reason, heroin became generally available, because the economic and social conditions are so different. Probably there normal people prefer to be stupefied rather than endure ordinary life. Similarly the reported evils of hashish in underdeveloped North African countries are probably only symptoms of poverty.

The moral question is perhaps slightly easier to attack. Here, of course, I am putting my personal views. My own feeling is that adults who know what they are doing – and no one can become a heroin addict without this knowledge – should be allowed to get on with it. I am not convinced that heroin use, in a sensible climate of opinion, is necessarily worse for the sort of person who finds it attractive than the vain attempt to live an ordinary life.

We should be humble enough to consider drug use one of the freedoms we enjoy in our society. And perhaps we forget that man is, almost above all his other qualities, a self-optimizing machine; that he is built to adapt to his training and surroundings in some way that tends to increase his chances for survival. Often his behaviour seems inconvenient, intolerable, self-destructive; this is because we can see only the half of the situation that lies outside the organism – the equally important internal arrangements of the drug user are hidden from us. We ought to consider the idea that in the situation he finds himself, his behaviour is more for his good than not. We should hesitate to interfere unless we can make radical changes either in his internal or external environments, or both, and so make drug use an option that he will prefer not to exercise.

These considerations apply particularly strongly to adolescent drug users. Addiction or habituation rather than occasional use is a symptom of something badly wrong. The fact that their personalities have not finally formed means there is some hope of altering them internally and externally enough to make drug use unnecessary; and we have an obvious duty to make this attempt. But it has to be well considered; superficial efforts may well exacerbate their problems.

Practical Considerations Relevant to Drug Control

One solution to a drug problem is to forget it. In the West, where the objective damage due directly to the use of drugs is small, much of the ultimate harm they do is caused by the reaction of hostile social attitudes. Thus in France, although the country was the international centre of the heroin traffic in the thirties and after, although heroin factories still exist round Marseilles, there are, officially, only sixty addicts and no drug problem. One suspects that this is simply due to the French tolerance for individual aberration. In the same way we have no barbiturate 'problem', although this drug is actually and potentially much more dangerous than heroin.

However, we are hardly likely to achieve such karmic acceptance. The opposite of acceptance is penal restriction of drug use, a policy pursued, apparently without great success, in the U.S.A., Canada, Hong Kong and other countries. In fact, as will appear below, this policy does actually reduce *addiction* – though unfortunately it produces more virulent side-effects. It is extremely important that we, in Britain, do not make this mistake. Not only can it cause misery, degradation, illness, squalor and early death in addicts, it is brutalizing for society, and because of its lack of overall success generates an extremist public attitude that makes more liberal approaches politically impossible. We have this problem in a mild way with marihuana now; the Americans, many of whom feel that the penal approach was a disastrous mistake, find it difficult now to experiment with more lenient methods.

The hard line towards addiction also tends to create and extrude intractable sub-cultures of users. This process of separation is examined by Wilkins[4] in terms of feedback loops. Briefly, his argument is that as a minority appears it begins to establish its own recognition symbols, values, ways of behaving which distinguish it from the main culture. If its activities are anti-social, pressure from the main will tend to isolate it and to deny its members access to the ordinary rewards of society. This is met by a negative reaction in the minority culture which re-intensifies its rebellion; so the loop rolls on. This analysis alone would suggest that sub-cultures must expand explosively: experience shows this is not the case. Wilkins, having provided a force of expansion in the sub-culture, does not appear to consider the countervailing pressures which society brings to bear on it. There seem to be two restraining forces: society's physical power to restrict, or make difficult, the sub-culture's activities, and in the ultimate resort, to kill all its members; secondly, the more immediate point that as the distance between the minor and major groups increases, so the number of new recruits abnormal enough to be willing to make the jump decreases. One sees the operation of this second control in the British Nazi Party whose members are few, but very extreme. The danger in applying pressure to the several sub-species of drug user is that we reduce the willingness of the compulsive drug user to accept our society and to accept help from it, and we make communication with him almost impossible. Extreme pressure, short of annihilation, simply produces a small number of absolutely intractable deviates: drug addiction in America shows this sort of position. By relaxing social pressure one runs the risk of increasing the numbers of people affected, but one also increases their accessibility. In the end we have probably gained. A second beneficial result is that as social pressure is reduced, so more diverse agencies can help with the problem. Extreme pressure calls for the Army, something less the police, less again and one can use doctors, social workers, psychiatrists. So many doctors in America have gone to prison for giving drugs to addicts in an attempt to establish a relationship with them that useful medical and psychiatric help is now almost unavailable to the drug user, except in the few rather isolated hospitals that deal with these cases.

Another consequence of using force to suppress drug use is an inconsistency that should be unacceptable in a civilized society. Drug users are recognized as being ill;* their illness is the cause of their drug use; therefore potential drug users are ill. The police are being used to repress symptoms of conditions that need medical attention.

International Control of Drugs

One of the first international organizations to reach within the frontiers of member states of the League of Nations, and now the United Nations, is the machinery that controls the manufacture and international trade in addictive drugs. As a piece of bureaucracy, it is impressive and serves as a valuable model for other international endeavours, such as the control of nuclear energy; as a method of preventing addiction and illicit drug use throughout the world, it is singularly ineffective.

A thorough account of its operation would be tedious. It is enough to say that in theory the member countries submit yearly estimates of their manufacture and consumption of some eighty dependence-producing drugs. An elaborate sum then shows what has gone astray; the nation responsible is invited to explain itself. The major defect of this system is that illicit manufacturers submit no estimates, and until 1961 no country was obliged to report its growth of poppy. Even now many countries where much poppy is grown have not the internal organization to make this report. In its broad effects the system of treaties, conferences and conventions has slowly driven the manufacture of heroin – the most compact opiate – back into the East, nearer to the poppy

*Or rather, they were. The first Brain Report regarded addiction as 'an expression of mental disorder rather than a form of criminal behaviour'. The second says that the addict is 'a sick person, provided he does not resort to criminal acts' when, presumably, he is no longer sick. (*Reports of the Interdepartmental Committee on Drug Addiction*, H.M.S.O., 1961, 1965.)

fields. But any successes in controlling addiction, such as Japan's or Formosa's before the war, are due to individual rather than collective effort.

This mechanism has only secondary effects in Britain. When the machinery was being constructed during the thirties, our domestic drug problem was negligible. We were able to accede to the most demanding treaties, and were glad to, both as an example to more indulgent nations, and so that we could apply the most rigorous standards in our own colonies. In particular we were anxious to repress a subversive Egyptian sub-culture that centred on hashish. It seems that but for the needs of empire, we would not have proscribed hashish, and we would now have no cannabis problem. Since our heroin problem is home-grown, and state-financed (directly attributable, with much of the rest of the world's addiction problems, to our refusal to let China ban opium in the 1830s, and to our Opium War victory of 1842), international control of drugs is irrelevant to our troubles. If, by some disaster of public policy, we allow a real black market to rise here, there is no reason to suppose that the United Nations Narcotics Commission will cause traffickers much difficulty in getting supplies from abroad.

Black Market

A practical and moral reason for preferring some sort of liberal drug control system, is to avoid the growth of a black market. It is no longer believed that a vigorous black market in itself makes addicts (see p. 34), but there are a number of more serious peripheral disadvantages. For one thing it occupies a number of people in work that serves no useful social purpose, and it occupies an equal number of more useful people in attempts to stop it. In fact, it is probably fair to say that in a vigorous situation of repression, the black marketeers and the police work in mutually unhelpful partnership. The black market provides the police with addicts and peddlers to arrest, seizures of drugs, and prestige; the police provide the traffickers with a captive market that cannot haggle or object, whose only price ceiling is set by their own abilities to steal, rob and whore. The black market too inadvertently helps the police combat addiction, for the drugs are sadly diluted at every stage of their journey. 'Cutting' a parcel of heroin in half only five times between grower and addict will reduce its purity to 3 per cent; its price will increase several hundred times over the journey. Thus an ounce of heroin that can be bought in Italy for $60 will fetch $28,000 on the streets of New York[5] – a happy commercial advantage the Mafia owes entirely to the energy of the American Department of the Treasury. The result of this dilution is that very few addicts, perhaps one in five, actually have had enough heroin to become addicted.[6]

Although an active black market reduces addiction and drug use, it does nothing to relieve the social damage due to the addict's way of life, and it also causes him to commit a great deal of expensive crime to support his habit. Winick estimates that each addict in New York has to steal up to $90,000 worth of goods a year.[5]

In the summer of 1969 there were rumours that a proper black market operation was being set up in London. Powdered heroin, either imported from China or made in France, was being found in police searches, and it was estimated[12] that some 40,000 fixes (enough to supply 300 addicts) were being smuggled into Britain every month. But by May 1970 Chinese heroin had almost disappeared. Perhaps the traffic had been suppressed by the Chinese community in Britain, who take very good care of their public relations. In any case, a black market can only develop against a system of repression: as long as addicts can get nearly enough heroin without much difficulty, there can be no solid opening for a black market in opiates.

It is a heartening sign of the success of the heroin containment strategy that the black market price of methadone, the slow-acting, unexciting opiate substituted in some treatments for heroin (see p. 149), has now risen to between 75p and £1 a grain. Two years ago it could hardly be given away.

Some of the vast mass of new research into drugs has been on the side of the user. An interesting project was analysis of drugs purchased on the street for fidelity to description and purity. A gross of drugs bought in Munich in 1972 showed only 80 that were as advertised; the other 64 samples were either adulterated or something completely different. One sample of LSD turned out to be 60 per cent sulphuric acid.[17] An agency exists in America for routine analysis of drug samples; useful as a guide to what is actually happening as well as providing material for the legal defence of drug users.

Police

One result of the explosive spread of drug use since 1965 has been the increased interest of the police. Many policemen now have experience of drug users, and find they pose an unfamiliar and unpleasant problem. The police are trained and organized to deal with professional criminals; both the police and criminal sub-culture have grown up together over the last century and a half. Both sides know the rules and have a certain respect for each other. With drug users the police are at a loss. These are people who offend all their instincts for order and discipline; while criminals provide an opponent one can decently dislike, young addicts can only be objects of pity. Yet society requires the police to track them down and arrest them as if they were criminals. The links between drug culture and the anti-authoritarianism of student politics, with the fact that many well-known and wealthy young people in the pop business, acting, films, are drug users, exacerbates the difficulties of the police, who dimly feel that their job of protecting society shouldn't include making available the freedom for this sort of self-indulgence. Terence Jones, a Detective Superintendent with the Hertfordshire Constabulary, neatly sums up the situation in his *Drugs and the Police*.[11]

The world of drug addiction is a strange one and one in which the police officer sometimes feels it difficult to mingle. Used as he is to the jargon of the criminal and his more predictable ways, the police officer finds the rather juvenile slang of the addict and his complete lack of direction rather nauseating. They are pitiful people so much in need of the help they spurn. They are dangerous people not only to themselves but to every impressionable young person with whom they come in contact. If they won't be cured they must be controlled. This is the role of the police.

The difficulty in police relationships with drug users is that, fundamentally, police forces are trained and organized to prevent one person doing something illegal to another person. There is always a victim/informant and a criminal. The police stand in the middle as an almost neutral agency, which must receive the complaint and information of the one before it can proceed against the other. Once that is done, it lapses into passivity again.*

When policemen have to deal with drug users, the situation is quite different. Here there is no complainant. The drug user is doing whatever is illegal to *himself*. In an attempt to manufacture the complainant police organization and training demands, they have to cast the user himself in this role – hence Jones writes: 'They are pitiful people so much in need of the help they spurn.' Not unnaturally, since they must conceive they are acting for the users' ultimate good, as 'complainant' the police tend to be rather arbitrary in their treatment of him in the criminal role. So when the Advisory Committee on Drug Dependence held its hearings on police powers,[13] 'Release' complained that the police had assumed arbitrarily wide powers of search, made it unnecessarily difficult for young prisoners to secure bail, made charges before the substance was analysed, and made it difficult or impossible for young prisoners to telephone parents or solicitors. The courts, too, are less than helpful: the two biggest magistrates' courts in central London do not, as a matter of principle, give legal aid in drugs cases. A thorough review of the practice of British policy and courts is to be found in *Guilty until Proved Innocent?*, an assessment of the Criminal Law Revision Committee's eleventh report: *Evidence (General)*.

Another interesting result of the lack of an 'injured party' in drug offences, is the lack of control over policemen who handle drugs, particularly in large quantities. In the ordinary crime – say of theft – there is an injured party who has lost goods or money. Even though the police – for their own profit – and the criminal, to minimize his punishment, might like to conceal some or all of the proceeds of the crime, the injured party will prevent this, because he wants his property back or insurance

*See my *Scotland Yard*, London, 1970, for a fuller analysis of this.

169

compensation for his full loss. But when a drugs trafficker is arrested with, let us say, a hundred-weight of hashish in his car, he is unlikely to complain if the police keep 109 lb for themselves, and charge him in court with possession of 1 lb. Thus it is easy and profitable for the police to become dealers in drugs themselves, through, of course, traffickers they have arrested, whom they can turn into accomplices through withholding their power to prosecute.

Having referred to some general points, we can now consider the control of different classes of drugs.

The Law

A new Act came into effect in 1973: the 'Misuse of Drugs Act 1971'. This consolidated the existing law, extended it and made it possible for new drugs to be added or dropped from the prohibited schedules by an Order in Council – that is, without reference to Parliament. Optimistic persons have seen in this an opening through which the Home Secretary could legalize cannabis without political scandal.

The new Act repeals the Dangerous Drugs Acts of 1965 and 1967, and the Drugs (Prevention of Misuse) Act 1964. It divides drugs into three classes: *A* includes opium, heroin, morphine, pethidine, cannabinol (not as a part of hashish or marihuana), LSD and other hallucinogens, injectable amphetamines, notably methedrine; *B* consists of codeine, pholcodeine, cannabis, cannabis resin, and five stimulant drugs of the amphetamine type, of which the three most important are: benzedrine, dexamphetamine, drinamyl; *C* contains lesser amphetamine-like drugs.

Penalties are related to the type of drug and the type of offence – possession or trafficking. The maximum penalty of fourteen years' imprisonment and/or an unlimited fine applies to the following acts to do with drugs in Classes A and B: producing; supplying or offering to supply; possessing with intent to supply to another; unlawfully importing or exporting; being the occupier of premises and knowingly permitting drugs transactions to take place there; and contravening a direction prohibiting a doctor from possessing, supplying or prescribing a controlled drug.

Simple possession of a Class A drug is punishable by seven years' imprisonment, Class B by five years, Class C by two years – and/ or an unlimited fine in all cases.

To stop over-prescribing, which seems to have been a cause of the rapid growth of heroin addiction in the last few years, the Act gives the Home Secretary power to ban any doctor from prescribing, supplying or possessing drugs in the three classes.

The Act creates two statutory defences to drugs charges. A defence to possession is to show an intention to dispose of the drug in a lawful manner. Although it's meant to cover people like schoolmasters who may confiscate drugs from their charges, and are therefore protected as long as they destroy them or give them to the police as soon as may be, it must also apply to anyone who, on being stopped by a policeman in the street, produces a joint and gives it to him, saying, 'I'm so glad to have met you; I was on my way to the police station to hand this in.' The second defence protects people charged with production, supply or possession who can prove that they didn't know, nor had reason to suspect the existence of a fact that the prosecution has to prove. So, if someone gave you some white powder saying it was bicarbonate of soda although it was heroin, you could escape conviction if you could convince a court of your mistake.

The new law also introduces the word 'knowingly' into the section which makes it illegal to permit drug transactions in your house. This is to avoid the problem of *Sweet* v. *Parsley*, where a Miss Sweet, who lent her cottage to some friends, was convicted under the old law when they were convicted of possession of cannabis although she wasn't there and knew nothing about it.

Apart from saying that the new law is as wrong as the old in treating drug use or abuse as a criminal act rather than a social preference or, in extreme cases, as a symptom of some major psychological problem, there is not a great deal to criticize. Rather more worrying is the development of case law after the successful prosecution of *Oz* in 1972 under the Obscene Publications Act. One of the passages complained of was a medical advice column called Dr Hip Pocrates – written in fact by the student health physician at Berkeley, California. An LSD user had written to say that his left hand and arm had gone totally dead during an LSD trip. Dr. Hip replied that:

All LSD available on the black market today is illegally produced by chemists who, of necessity, run make-shift laboratories. Compounds produced in these laboratories contain impurities which may be more dangerous than the pure drugs.

LSD is related to ergot, a substance which causes constriction of blood vessels including those in the brain. Ergot is a fungus which grows on rye and other grains. During the Middle Ages epidemics of ergot poisoning occurred in which the characteristic symptoms were gangrene the feet, legs, hands and arms.

If I were you I would have a thorough physical examination. You live near a Free Clinic where you can speak frankly to a physician about these experiences.[18]

The prosecution successfully contended that since there was no explicit advice not to use LSD except under medical supervision, the passage was obscene.

Control

We must assume for the moment that we should do all we can to prevent people, particularly adolescents, developing the heroin habit.

The present theory of control is elegant, and if it could be made to work, foolproof. The essence is that each addict is given free exactly as much as his body needs for the next day. He has no option but to inject it; there is none over to make new addicts, eventually he and all the other existing addicts will give up drugs or die. Since supply is exactly fitted to demand, there is no cause for a black market, and therefore no generation of new addicts in that quarter. End of problem. In practice it is not quite like that. The quantity of heroin supplied is critical: too little creates a black market by demand, too much creates one by supply. That every two addicts recruit a third every year (see above p. 20) shows the extent of this over-supply in the past. This second state of affairs contributed to the addict explosion that faces us now, a situation caused as much by a breakdown in medical services as by the new habit of proselytizing. There are only a few doctors who are prepared to put up with addicts – perhaps only a dozen in London, and hardly any in the provinces. As the number of addicts increased, these practitioners became flooded with customers, were quite unable to form the close, authoritative parental bonds with each of their patients that successful control or treatment demands, and simply to make their lives bearable were forced to prescribe lavishly. With no workable system of identification, addicts were able to go to two or three doctors and get treble rations; with no means of withdrawing patients these doctors were unable to establish proper dose levels. Consultations became horse-trading sessions at which the addict and the doctor tried to outwit each other: since the addict has one mania, but the doctor several hundred things to think about, the issue was hardly in doubt. At least one doctor seems to have been won over, for he was described to me by some of his patients as forcing heroin on them. The Brain Committee were told of one case of a boy who had jabbed his arm with a pin, and then succeeded in getting a prescription. Under these conditions our system could hardly be expected to work.

In a series of interviews with doctors who treat addicts, one told the *Sunday Times*

. . . every interview with an addict is a battle of wills. They are driven by a need one can't understand oneself, and they will lie, beg and scheme to get more, and more again.

Another doctor:

Sometimes you get tired of arguing and think, 'Oh well, what's the harm?' And you let whoever it is have the extra grain, or half grain. But, you see, if it isn't making you tired, you're not doing your job.[7]

In the absence of facilities for withdrawal, or a simple chemical test to establish the addict's dosage, the only way society can keep the amount of heroin prescribed to the amount that is physiologically needed is by using doctors who have the energy to force addicts back to the sticking point in debate.

One immediate remedy would be to increase the amount of will-power opposing addicts' demands by recruiting more doctors to deal with them. Say there are a thousand addicts, and that the most one doctor can handle adequately is 30 – that gives a requirement of 33 doctors, 21 more than the dozen already practising. If we are to take addiction seriously, these doctors had better work full-time at the problem, perhaps under contract to a central body that would also be responsible for hospitalization, psychiatric and social after-care services, registration of addicts and research into addiction. In terms of employment, comparing these doctors with general practitioners, we are saying that each addict needs as much attention as a hundred people on an ordinary panel. Considering the demands addicts make, this is reasonable.

The Brain Committee's Second Report proposed that the prescription of heroin should be confined to Treatment Centres, and suggested that there should be a power to detain addicts who have volunteered for withdrawal while they pass the crisis. Some of this Report's proposals were put into action in April 1968. It then became illegal for any doctor, not specially licensed by the Ministry of Health, to prescribe heroin and cocaine to addicts. Some 600 licences were granted to doctors working in those hospitals who had, or were likely to set up Treatment Centres. So far there are twenty-six in London, a couple in Birmingham, Manchester and so on. The aim at the time of writing seems not to be so much directed towards treatment as controlling the prescription of heroin. An addict, once he is 'registered' at a Treatment Centre – the details are relayed to a file at the Home Office – then has to attend once a week. A prescription for the drugs he needs is posted to his chosen chemist every week, and he goes there every day to pick up the next day's supply. The essence of the scheme is uniformity of treatment: once a dose is settled the addict has to stick to it, and if he goes to another Treatment Centre the doctor there will discover his dose and prescribe the same. The result is that (a) whatever the addict's original dose was his tolerance soon builds up to what he is getting and therefore (b) he has none to spare for the black market but (c) he is not 'hungry' enough to buy extra drugs. In recent years the British treatment system has followed the American pattern in converting heroin addicts to methadone (see p. 148), a much less dynamic drug, and one that is much less susceptible to black-market operations.

So far the doctors involved in the programme are feeling their way. At least the total addict population is being revealed and there is some regular contact between them and the State. It is interesting that some doctors complain that because the 'Treatment Centre system' says how much drugs each addict should be given, it destroys the 'doctor-patient relationship'. This is true, but perhaps it is because the doctor-patient relationship is irrelevant in the drug addiction problem. The classical relationship between the two is based on the idea of a single disease; the two collaborate to defeat it, and no one else has any authority in the matter. If the disease is easily communicated it may establish an epidemic, and society as a whole has to be represented – the patient's contacts have to be traced, he has to be put in a special hospital, etc. With heroin addiction, the problem is, as it were, *all* epidemic and no disease. It now appears to have been something of a fallacy to treat it as if it were a disease because the 'germs' – the doses of heroin – are social currency, they are given, sold, traded, passed about in response to social rather than biological laws. In order to control heroin addiction, society, and that means that doctors who deal with addicts, has to present a united face. It is no use one having a 'hard' attitude and another 'soft'. Both may be equally successful with diseases and patients that cannot move about, but in the drug situation all the 'hard' doctors' patients leave and go to the 'soft' ones.

In perspective, the 1968 moves to control heroin by the limitation of the right to prescribe heroin and cocaine to addicts was as much aimed at doctors as at addicts themselves, because it had become apparent that the medical profession itself was unable to control those of its members who, for one reason or another, prescribed irresponsibly.

An example of this was the unfortunate affair of Dr Petro. This elderly practitioner had, for what reasons it does not matter, a very soft attitude towards drug addicts. He ran an extraordinarily rickety practice round Paddington from 1966 to 1968, seeing his patients in station waiting-rooms, hotels, wherever he happened to be. He was widely criticized for 'selling' prescriptions for heroin, but since he didn't work for the Health Service he could only live by charging fees. He was investigated by the General Medical Council and struck off the register for infamous professional practice, though the fault was probably not so much his, as society's inability to deal with the addicts who flocked to him. One can also criticize the enforcement of medical ethics, for although his practice was disapproved of little could be done to control him short of the final, blasting step of disqualification. The Misuse of Drugs Act, 1971 (see p. 178) gives the Home Secretary the power to remove a doctor's right to prescribe certain classes of drugs.

Well-intentioned though the Treatment Centres may have been, their operation has come under some criticism. Cutbacks in funding caused by the economic difficulties of the late seventies have reduced the scope of their action. According to a *Release* report[19] published in 1977, it was becoming harder to register at a clinic – at best the paperwork might take two to three weeks, or, at worst, so long that the addict gave up and went elsewhere. Admission to hospital for a physical cure took even longer, while the necessary follow-up services needed to reform the ex-addict's lifestyle, which, as we have seen, are much more important than 'cure', have been almost completely abandoned.

Barbiturate

Although this drug is objectively as addictive as and rather more destructive than heroin, it is at the moment controlled only under the Pharmacy and Poisons Act. As a Fourth Schedule drug, it can only be sold retail on a prescription given by a doctor, dentist or vet. It would seem logical to make it a D.D.A. drug, but although the public in general is very willing to follow the lead of authority in its attitude to drugs, there must be so many people more or less dependent on barbiturates that sudden restrictive measures would simply make vast numbers of outlaws. Besides, in the sense that there is very little *worry* about the drug, we have no barbiturate problem; there is little point in creating one by legislation. A Campaign on Use and Restriction of Barbiturates (CURB) was started in the autumn of 1975[20] to persuade doctors – mainly by direct-mail propaganda – to reduce their prescribing of this most damaging drug, which is responsible for most U.K. admissions to mental hospitals for drug dependence. It is hoped that by 1978 there will have been a substantial reduction in the use of barbiturates.

Amphetamines

Assuming that it is impossible to stop people taking some sort of mood and personality alterers, amphetamines in moderate doses are probably as good as alcohol, and in some respects better, especially for the young. There would be little objection to teenagers taking half a dozen or so over a week-end; but the habit of swallowing the pills in handfuls is alarming. These excesses, if persistent, are symptoms of personality disorder, but they can also occur in those who have not yet learned, and are not taught by the existing sub-culture, how to use the drug properly. There are perhaps two things to be done about this.

The first is to alter the attitudes of adults towards this drug. While parents and teachers regard it as the purple kiss of Satan, teenage attitudes to it are hardly likely to be more rational. If a boy takes the pills to be rebellious and because he wants to shock, he has no reason to limit his dose. They are not, to him, an ordinary substance like tea or food or beer; they have a symbolic value and the more he takes the more emancipated he becomes. We can short-circuit this problem by bringing to bear the same attitudes as we do towards teenage drinking; to say that it is silly and unpleasant to take too much.

Then, it is unrealistic to expect to stamp out the supply of amphetamines. People all over the world like them too much; the prospects for repression are shown by their ready availability in H.M. prisons,[8] and the failure of a recent campaign to stamp them out in Sweden.

The ideal would be to dilute amphetamine preparations as we do alcohol; this however is likely to be impossible because of the cost of storing and transporting the vast quantities that are used in medicine. It might be more practical to include a substance that would cause nausea if twice the maximum clinical dose were taken. It would be necessary to make these 'safe' pills available to the black market in some subtle way, so their abundance would drive out unsafe foreign imports.

It will still be necessary to nurture a sensible and acceptable cultural attitude towards the use of amphetamines. For this reason legal sanctions will still be necessary, but the efforts of the police and the courts should be directed less towards the futile task of eliminating them than to the repression of unacceptable social behaviour under their influence. People who use amphetamines must be taught that they have to behave as responsibly as alcohol drinkers. That is, after all, not a very high standard.

The Drugs (Prevention of Misuse) Act, 1964, prohibits the importation or manufacture of amphetamines without a licence from the Home Secretary and provides penalties for the illegal possession of the drug: a fine of £200 and/or six months imprisonment on summary conviction, or an unspecified fine and/or imprisonment for two years on conviction or indictment. It has been repealed and replaced by the relevant sections of The Misuse of Drugs Act 1971, which imposes heavier penalties. It cannot be said that either Act represents very imaginative or effective legislation.

A more practical step was taken in October 1968 when the Ministry of Health persuaded the manufacturers of methedrine, the potent, liquid form of amphetamine, to supply it only to hospitals for a trial period of a year. This was done because the institution of Treatment Centres, and the consequent beginnings of control over heroin, had multiplied addicts' use of methedrine some five times in a few months. By 1977 prescribing of amphetamines had almost stopped, largely as a result of initiatives taken by doctors themselves.

Cannabis

Black market hashish in Britain is supplied either by well-organized smuggling, often in large parcels, of hemp grown in the Lebanon, Pakistan or Cyprus, or by 'do it yourself' smuggling by students and young people who have been abroad on holiday. This last, as the Advisory Committee on Drug Dependence reported,[15] has stabilized the black market and made it unattractive to really large-scale criminal operators. There is evidence that the use of cannabis is steadily spreading over the country. Seizures of imports by the Customs have smoothly increased since the war, and the numbers of cannabis prosecutions have also increased, with white people being convicted more often than coloured since 1964. A little hemp is grown in Britain, but the climate does not really suit the plant.

Possibly because of the widespread association of marihuana use with holding radical political opinions, governments seem prepared to spend considerable sums of money on scientific aid for attacking it. Thus the Americans have developed an airborne 'sniffer' that can detect fields of hemp from a height of 200-300 feet – these devices were used in Mexico during the 1970 campaign to eliminate the traffic into the U.S.A. In England the Atomic Weapons Research Establishment at Aldermaston has produced a technique for detecting cannabinol condensates on the fingers of smokers for up to three hours after smoking, with a guaranteed minimum time of detection of one hour. It is said that washing with soap and water affords no protection, but it is possible that washing in ether would, since this is the agent used to transfer the residues to the chromatographic apparatus.[15]

There are no apparent reasons for cannabis's status as a Dangerous Drug. It is not addictive, its use does not in Western society cause crime or unacceptable sexuality, and it does not lead to addiction to the hard drugs. The major problem with this drug is that it is illegal. This has three undesirable effects: first, an underground, cannabis-using sub-culture is created and maintained that puts the potential heroin addict one step nearer access to the hard drugs; second, it lessens respect for D.D.A. drugs in the thousands of young people who have tried marihuana or hashish and know from personal experience how harmless the drug is; third, it causes considerable waste of man-power, either through creative and educated people being sent to prison for possession of the drug – a Glasgow doctor was sentenced to six months recently – or through the use of policemen, who would be better otherwise employed, to track down the drug and its users.

The non-addictiveness of cannabis, and the dependence of the smoker's experiences on what he learns from the sub-group that uses the drug, mean that it is possible for society to control the behaviour of users. After nearly forty years of repression most of the rowdiness has been eliminated from cannabis-using groups in this country, and it seems that the behaviour of the users of this drug could now quite adequately be controlled by the ordinary machinery of the law. Legalization of cannabis – as the *Lancet*[9] pointed out – would offer considerable revenue in taxation. My own impression is that the Home Office would be happy to be quit of this problem – except that legalization of cannabis would be the political suicide of the incumbent Home Secretary; but Britain is restrained by the international agreements that proscribe this drug along with the opiates and cocaine.

Since 1966 things have moved fast in the cannabis field. Large numbers of people use the drug – the Advisory Committee on Drug Dependence, quoted on p. 83, accepted that there are 30,000–300,000 users, and a survey done for the B.B.C. TV programme *Midweek* in 1973 showed that four million people in Britain had smoked cannabis. Public opinion, from its relatively uninformed state in the mid sixties, is becoming sharply polarized. In the meantime the salient events were: the trial of the Rolling Stones in 1967 for possession of cannabis, the publication of the well-known full-page advertisement in *The Times*, paid for by the Beatles, which began with the statement, 'The law against marijuana is immoral in principle and unworkable in practice' and went on to set out the current medical view of the drug – much as it is put in these pages. It drew attention to the disproportionately heavy sentences available for those convicted of possessing the drug – ten years imprisonment or a fine of £1,000 – and was signed by some sixty respectable names from science, medicine and the more up-to-date arts. An organization, 'Release', was formed to organize legal advice for young people arrested on drugs charges; run by young people itself, it serves as a useful link between the world of drugs and the world of the establishment. The Wootton Committee reported, late 1968, in the sense that marihuana was not a dangerous drug, and that while the penalties for possessing small quantities of it should be nominal or abolished, the penalties for trafficking in it should be made heavier. In effect this would begin to bring the law on marihuana into line with that on alcohol. The next step would be for the State to make marihuana preparations available through selected, controlled outlets. But this is not likely to happen for some years, if only because licit marihuana would pose an enormous threat to the equally enormous established cigarette and alcohol industries. A threat to them is a threat to the State, because a third of the British government's income is derived from taxes levied on the sale of these addictive drugs. Non-addictive marihuana might prove an unreliable substitute. But nevertheless one hears that the major cigarette companies have already completed marketing studies; they have designed packs and registered trade names for a marihuana marketing operation. At the same time the alcohol manufacturers in America, and probably in Britain, are spending large sums – of the order of $100 million a year – to 'de-advertise' marihuana, by financing critical scientific studies, and by subsidizing anti-drug politicians.

On the other hand the police, as so often when they are asked to enforce unpopular laws with which they themselves agree, have found themselves in sharper and sharper opposition to public opinion over this question. This is one example of the police–public dichotomy: the police see and deal with only the squalor of drug addiction; to them all drug use is pernicious and crippling. Because the police tidy these people so neatly away the public – particularly the intellectual pro-marihuana public – doesn't see them. While both sides think they are arguing the same topic, they work from contradictory premises to reach opposite conclusions. Anyway, at the time of writing the police have the last laugh. Marihuana prosecutions are very frequent, and as often happens when the police are put in a situation they dislike, they take the letter of the law to extreme lengths. An example was the recent prosecution of no less than seventeen people at the Old Bailey for possession of one small lump of hashish found in a guitar case in the same room. (In another charge, which one has to admire as a stroke of jurisprudential genius, three heroin addicts playing around with their works in the bathroom of the same flat, were charged with an obscene exhibition. But the judge directed the jury to return a verdict of not guilty on this last charge.)

A survey by *Release*[21] of sentencing policy in courts in England and Wales reviewed 1974 figures. In that year there were nearly 10,000 successful prosecutions for cannabis offences. One fifth resulted in prison sentences, either immediate or suspended. Simple possession was usually punished with fines ranging from £40 to £70, though in some out-of-the-way places where magistrates were not used to the offence, they could be as high as £75 to £100. Couriers of drugs in bulk got roughly one to three years, while dealers in large quantities for profit got up to six years.

Hallucinogens

These drugs present the same problems as amphetamines, only in a more acute form. Their ease of manufacture and concealment means that extirpation is impossible,* while the immaturity of the LSD-using community offers no guarantees that the drug will be used responsibly. It is necessary that something be done because, although the psychosis rate among normals is low, illicit LSD use is likely to produce psychosis more frequently. The drug is apt to be taken in hostile or worrying situations, and illicit use tends to attract people who are already unstable. Since this psychosis can cause a long illness, it is desirable to be more stringent over the control of hallucinogens than the raw accident rates would suggest.

In terms of law enforcement, there is almost nothing that can be done. Since LSD is such a concentrated drug, large amounts can easily be smuggled into the country, or concealed when it is here. The Customs can only hope to seize imports if they are tipped off, and the police can only hope to discover illicit labora-

*In spite of the illegality of LSD in America it is estimated that 10,000 students in the University of California have tried it.[10]

tories on the basis of 'information received'. In fact, in 1969 and 1970, several such laboratories were found as a result of normal underworld treachery, but this activity can have had little effect on the market supply of LSD. There were also reports that large quantities were originating from the chemistry department of the Humboldt University in East Berlin, and that the raw materials for manufacturing LSD here were supplied, with Government connivance, from East Germany, as part of yet another sinister Communist plot to corrupt the youth of the West. An interesting study of the purity of black market drugs in Canada [16] found that only 68 per cent of samples alleged to contain LSD actually did so, and that only half consisted of the pure drug. It is significant for the British drug user that in general British LSD is considered inferior to that of North American manufacture, so one might suppose a similar study here would show even more startling results.

So the only practicable control on the use of LSD is in the attitude of drug users themselves. Perhaps happily, the first proselytizing enthusiasms of the mid sixties seem to be waning. Certainly LSD psychiatric casualties are becoming rarer.

Cocaine

As this edition was going to press in the early summer of 1974, a wave of cocaine use (see p. 86) was spreading over the underground communities of London. Unknown as an illicit drug in England since the naughty twenties, its use may be forced on those who normally smoke marihuana by the success of the concerted campaign against cannabis by the customs and law enforcement agencies of the West. By 1977 cocaine had become quite fashionable, but its expense restricted its use to small and rather self-admiring circles.

Finally

We should try to see drug use as an inevitable result of technical advance. There are few people so satisfied with their lives that they will refuse any alteration. It is unrealistic to expect them to, more unrealistic to see this always as some sort of sickness. It is perfectly within man's power to develop sensible attitudes to all drugs; to use them rather than be used by them. At the same time we must not expect perfectibility. As the major social ills are cleared away so minor ones emerge; drug abuse is one of them that may, by the time the situation is stabilized, affect 50,000–70,000 people in this country. Drug problems are the price we must pay for having effective medicines.

As a corollary to this, we must remember that the availability or attractiveness of drugs seems to play a small part in the formation of drug dependent personalities. Almost without exception, the studies quoted here of people who become unable to live without drugs of one sort or another – some addictive, some not – show that the decisive causes of this situation lie in their personalities and not in the drug. Drug dependence is a symptom and not a disease.

References

1 The Meaning of Drug

1 *W.H.O. Technical Report Series 287*, 1964, p. 5
2 Wikler, A., *Psychiatric Quarterly*, 26, 1952, p. 270
3 Sargant, W., *Battle for the Mind*, Heinemann, London, 1957
4 National Council on Alcoholism
5 R.O.S.P.A., *Road Accidents Statistical Review*, 3, no. 15, Nov. 1965
6 Chief Constable of Glasgow, *Report*, 1964
7 *Statistical Review of Press and T.V. Advertising*, 33, no. 4, Oct–Nov. 1965, p. 58
8 Seebohm Rowntree, B., and Lavers, G. R., *English Life and Leisure*, Longmans, 1951
9 *Alcoholic Abuse*, Office of Health Economics, London, 1970
10 *Journal*, The Addiction Research Foundation, Toronto, 1 Oct. 1976

2 Archetypal Heroin

1 *Drug Addiction*, Report of the Interdepartmental Committee, H.M.S.O., 1961
2 Lindesmith, A. R., *Opiate Addiction*, Principia Press, Indiana, 1947
3 Zinberg, N. E., and Lewis, D. C., *New England Journal of Medicine*, 270, 1964, pp. 989 and 1045
4 Bewley, T., *British Medical Journal*, no. 2, 1965, p. 1284
5 Laurie, P., *Teenage Revolution*, Blond, London, 1965
6 Wikler, A., *Mechanisms of Action of Opiates and Opiate Antagonists* (U.S. Public Health Monograph 52)
7 Nyswander, Marie, *The Drug Addict as a Patient*, Grune & Stratton, New York, 1956
8 Hoffman, M., *Comprehensive Psychology*, 5, 1964, p. 262
9 Chein, I., *et al.*, *Narcotics, Delinquency and Social Policy*, Tavistock, London, 1964
10 Kolb, L., *Mental Hygiene*, 9, 1925, p. 699
11 De Ropp, R. S., *Drugs and the Mind*, Gollancz, London, 1958
12 Quoted by Nyswander, op. cit. ref. 7 above
13 Leong, E., Way, T., and Adler, K., *Pharmacological Review*, 12, 1960, p. 383
14 Hill, H. E., Belleville, R. E., and Wikler, A., *Archives of Neurology and Psychiatry*, 77, 1957, p. 28
15 Collier, H. O. J., *Nature*, 205, 1965, p. 181

REFERENCES

16 Schaumann, O., *Angewandte Chemie, 66*, 1954, p. 765

17 Spragg, S. D. S., *Morphine Addiction in Chimpanzees*, Comparative Psychology Monographs, Vol. 15, no. 7, 1940, p. 1

18 Ball, J. C., *Journal of Criminal Law, Criminology and Police Science, 56, no. 2*, 1965, p. 203

19 Kolb, L., *Archives of Neurology and Psychiatry, 20*, 1928, p. 171

20 Terry, C. E., and Pellens, Mildred, *The Opium Problem*, Commission on Drug Addictions, 1928 (U.S.A.)

21 Pescor, M. J., *U.S. Public Health Services Report, 24* (supp. 143), 1943

22 *Facts Concerning the U.S. Public Health Service Hospital, Lexington*, U.S. Department of Health Education and Welfare, 1965

23 Ball, J. C., and Cottrell, Emily S., *U.S. Public Health Reports, 80*, 1965, p. 471

24 Gerard, D. L., and Kornetsky, C., *Psychiatry Quarterly, 29*, 1955, p. 457

25 *Medindex, 2*, 1966, p. 107

26 Nelson, A. S., *International Journal of the Addictions*, Jan. 1966, p. 50

27 Kevaler-Menachem, F., Symposium of Study for Study of Addiction, New York, 1967

28 O'Donnell, J. A., *American Journal of Orthopsychology, 34, no. 5*, 1964, p. 948

29 Winick, C., *U.N. Bulletin on Narcotics*, Jan.–Mar. 1962

30 Bewley, T. H., *British Medical Journal, i*, 1968, p. 725

31 de Alarcón, R., and Rathod, N. H., *British Medical Journal, ii*, 1968, p. 549

32 Zacune, J., *et al.*, *International Journal of the Addictions, 4*, Dec. 1969, p. 557

33 *Report to the United Nations by Her Majesty's Government in the United Kingdom and Northern Ireland on the Working of the International Treaties on Narcotic Drugs for 1969*, Home Office, London, 1970

34 de Alarcón, R., *Bulletin on Narcotics, 21*, no. 3, July–Sept. 1969, p. 17

35 Monograph Series A, No. 2, Executive Office of the President, Special Action Office for Drug Abuse Prevention, May 1974

3 The Psychology of the Addict

1 Winick, C., *Law and Contemporary Problems, 22*, 1957, p. 9

2 Nyswander, Marie, *The Drug Addict as a Patient*, Grune & Stratton, New York, 1956

3 Carstairs, G. M., *Quarterly Journal of Studies on Alcohol, 15*, 1954, p. 220

4 Chein, I., *et al.*, *Narcotics, Delinquency and Social Policy*, Tavistock, London, 1964

5 Vaillant, G. E., *American Journal of Psychiatry, 122, no. 7*, 1966, p. 727

6 *Narcotic Drug Addiction*, U.S. Public Health Service Publication 1021

7 Frankau, Lady, *Canadian Medical Association Journal, 90*, 1964, p. 421

8 Lyle, D., *Esquire*, *65, no. 3*, March 1966

9 Hoffman, M., *Comprehensive Psychology*, *5*, 1964, p. 262

10 Wikler, A., *Psychiatric Quarterly*, *26*, 1952, p. 270

11 Carlson, E. T., and Simpson, M. M., *American Journal of Psychiatry*, *120*, 1963, p. 112

12 Wikler, A., *Mechanisms of Action of Opiates and Opiate Antagonists* (U.S. Public Health Monograph 52)

13 Laing, R. D., *The Divided Self*, Tavistock, London, 1960; Penguin Books, 1965

14 Wikler, A., *et al.*, *Psychopharmacologia*, *5*, 1963, p. 55

15 Beach, H. D., *Canadian Journal of Psychology*, *11*, 1957, p. 104

16 Davis, W. M., and Nichols, J. R., *Psychopharmacologia*, *3*, 1962, p. 139

17 Nichols, J. R., Headlee, C. P., and Coppock, H. W. J., *American Pharmacological Association* (Scientific Edition), *45*, 1956, p. 788

18 Albury, S., unpublished M.A. thesis, University of Sussex, 1968

4 Attitudes to Opiates

1 Williams, Clarence, *Jerry the Junker* (gramophone record), Black and White Records, 1934

2 Kerouac, J., *On the Road*, André Deutsch, London, 1958

3 Zinberg, N. E., and Lewis, D. C., *New England Journal of Medicine*, *270*, 1964, pp. 989 and 1045

4 Lyle, D., *Esquire*, *65, no. 3*, March 1966

5 Trocchi, A., *Cain's Book*, Calder, London, 1963

6 *The Times*, 21 Dec. 1965

7 *News of the World*, 18 Nov. 1962

8 *The Times*, 12 April 1965

9 *Sketch*, 13 Dec. 1965

5 Sleepers

1 Communication from Home Office, Narcotics Branch, 26.8.66

2 Editorial, *Lancet*, *ii*, 1954, p. 75

3 Editorial, *British Medical Journal*, *ii*, 1954, p. 1534

4 Hamburger, E., *Journal of the American Medical Association*, *189*, 1964, p. 366

5 Fraser, H. F., Wikler, A., and Essig, C. F., *Journal of the American Medical Association*, *166*, 1958, p. 126

6 *Medindex*, *2*, 1966

7 Freud, S., *Beyond the Pleasure Principle*, *Collected Papers*, International Psychoanalytic Press, New York, 1950

8 Eysenck, H. J., *Crime and Personality*, Routledge & Kegan Paul, London, 1964

9 Isbell, H., *Medical Clinics of North America*, *34, no. 2*, 1950, p. 425

REFERENCES

10 Trocchi, A., *Cain's Book*, Calder, London, 1963

11 Locket, S., *British Journal of Addiction*, *53*, 1957, p. 105

12 Hunter, R. A., *British Journal of Addiction*, *53*, 1957, p. 93

13 Hunter, R. A., and Greenberg, H. P., *Lancet*, *ii*, 1954, p. 58

14 Sargant, W., *Proceedings of the Royal Society of Medicine*, *51*, 1958, p. 353

15 Glatt, M. M., *U.N. Bulletin on Narcotics*, April–June, 1962

16 Kessel, N., and Walton, H., *Alcoholism*, Penguin Books, London, 1965

17 *Annual Report of the Ministry of Health* (Cmnd 2688), H.M.S.O., 1969

18 Smart, R. G., Schmidt, W., and Bateman, K., *Journal of Safety Research*, *I, no. 2*, June 1969, p. 67

19 Camps, F., and Robinson, A. E., *British Medical Journal*, 11 July 1970

6 Speed

1 *Medindex*, *2*, 1966

2 Sargant, W., and Blackburn, J. M., *Lancet*, *ii*, 1936, p. 1385

3 Bett, W. R., Howells, L. H., Macdonald, A. D., *Amphetamine in Clinical Medicine*, E. & S. Livingstone, Edinburgh, 1955

4 Eysenck, H. J., *Crime and Personality*, Routledge & Kegan Paul, London, 1964

5 Lindsley, D., and Henry, C. E., *Psychosomatic Medicine*, *4*, 1942, p. 140

6 Oswald, I., and Thacore, V. R., *British Medical Journal*, *ii*, 1963, p. 427

7 Sharpley, Anne, *Evening Standard*, 4 Feb. 1964

8 Sharpley, Anne, *Evening Standard*, 3 Feb. 1964

9 Prys Williams, G., *Decade of Drunkenness*, Christian Economic and Social Research Foundation, London, 1965

10 Sargant, W., *Battle for the Mind*, Heinemann, London, 1957

11 Scott, P. D., and Willcox, D. R. C., *see Lancet*, *ii*, 1964, p. 452

12 Howard, D. L., *Marriage Guidance*, Jan. 1966

13 Interview with Cmdr Millen, Metropolitan Police

14 Connell, P. H., *Amphetamine Psychosis*, Chapman & Hall, London, 1958

15 Connell, P. H., *Proceedings of the Leeds Symposium on Behavioural Disorders*, May & Baker Ltd, Dagenham, 1965

16 *Prison and Borstal After-care*, Annual Report of the Council of the Central After-care Association, H.M.S.O., 1963

17 Bell, D. S., and Trethowan, W. H., *Archives of General Psychiatry*, *4*, 1961, p. 74

18 Bell, D. S., and Trethowan, W. H., *Journal of Nervous and Mental Diseases*, *133*, 1961, p. 489

19 Parker, T., *Five Women*, Hutchinson, London, 1965

20 *Annual Report of the Ministry of Health* (Cmnd 2688), H.M.S.O., 1965, and communication from Home Office

21 Kiloh, L. G., and Brandon, S., *British Medical Journal*, *ii*, 1962, p. 40
22 *Registrar General's Statistical Review of England and Wales*, H.M.S.O., 1963
23 *Daily Mail*, 20 June 1962
24 *The Times*, 21 Feb. 1966
25 Wilson, C. W. M., and Beacon, S., *British Journal of Addiction*, *60*, 1964, p. 81

7 The Weed

1 Murphy, H. B. M., *U.N. Bulletin on Narcotics*, Jan.–Mar. 1963
2 Michaux, H., *Light Through Darkness*, trans. Chevalier, Orion Press, New York, 1963
3 Gautier, T., *Le Club des Haschischiens*, Feuilleton de la Presse Médicale, 10, VII, Paris, 1843
4 Baudelaire, C., *Les Paradis Artificiels*, trans. Symons, The Casanova Society, London, 1925
5 Ames, F., *Journal of Mental Science*, *104*, 1958, p. 972
6 Williams, E. G., *et al.*, *U.S. Public Health Report*, *61*, 1946, p. 1059
7 Adams, R., *Bulletins of the New York Academy of Medicine*, *18*, 1942, p. 705
8 *See* Martinec, R., and Felkova, M., *Pharmazie*, *14*, 1959, p. 276
9 Editorial, *Lancet*, *ii*, 1963, p. 989
10 Laing, R. D., *Sigma*, *6*, p. 7
11 *American Journal of Political Science*, *2*, 1931, p. 252
12 *Physical Culture*, *77*, 18 Feb. 1937
13 *Radio Stars*, 8 July 1938
14 Bigard, Barney, *Sweet Marihuana Brown* (gramophone record), Black and White Records, 1945
15 Johnson, D. McI., *Indian Hemp, a Social Menace*, Johnson, London, 1952
16 Ralph, J., *Sunday Graphic*, 16 and 23 Sept. 1951
17 Siler, J. F., *et al.*, *The Military Surgeon*, *73*, 1933, p. 269
18 Marcovitz, E., and Myers, H. J., *War Medicine*, *6*, 1944, p. 382
19 *The Marihuana Problem in the City of New York; Sociological, Medical, Psychological and Pharmacological Studies*, Cattell Press, Lancaster, Pa., 1944
20 Anslinger, H. J., and Tomkins, W. F., *The Traffic in Narcotics*, Funk & Wagnalls, New York, 1953
21 Bromberg, W., *Journal of the American Medical Association*, *113*, 1939, p. 4
22 Bromberg, W., *American Journal of Psychiatry*, *91*, 1934, p. 302
23 Meseinger, cited by Winick, see ref. 24 below
24 Winick, C., 'Marihuana Use by Young People', in *Drug Addiction in Youth*, ed. Harms, Pergamon, Oxford, 1965

REFERENCES

25 Chopra, R. N. and G. S., *Indian Medical Research Memoirs, 31*, July 1939

26 Allentuck, S., and Bowman, K. M., *American Journal of Psychiatry, 99*, 1942, p. 248

27 Lambo, T. A., *U.N. Bulletin on Narcotics*, Jan.–Mar. 1965

28 Becker, H. S., *American Journal of Sociology, 59*, 1953, p. 235

29 *Sunday Times*, 16 May 1965

30 *Cannabis*, Report by the Advisory Committee on Drug Dependence, H.M.S.O., 1969

31 *Interim Report of Commission of Enquiry into the Non-Medical Use of Drugs*, Queen's Printer for Canada, 1970, Penguin Books, 1972

32 Hindmarsh, I., *British Journal of Addiction, 64*, 1970, p. 395

33 *Daily Mirror*, 20 July 1970

34 Tennant, F. S., *et al.*, *Archives of General Psychiatry, 27*, July 1972

35 *New Scientist*, 8 June, 1972

36 Miles, C. G., *et al.*, Thirtieth International Congress on Alcoholism and Drug Dependence

37 *Drugs and Society, 2*, No. 12, Sept. 1973

38 *Journal*, The Addiction Research Foundation, Toronto, 1 Nov. 1975

8   Hallucinogens

1 Cohen, S., *Drugs of Hallucination*, Secker & Warburg, London, 1965

2 Rinaldi, F., and Himwich, H. E., *Science, 122*, 1955, p. 198

3 Klee, G. D., *Archives of General Psychiatry, 8*, 1963, p. 461.

4 Rosenthal, S. H., *American Journal of Psychiatry, 121*, 1964–5, p. 238

5 Klee, G. D., and Weintraub, W., in *Neuropsychopharmacology* (ed. Bradley, Deniker, Radouco-Thomas), Princeton, 1959, p. 457

6 Osmond, H., and Smythie, J. R., *Journal of Mental Science, 98*, 1952, p. 309

7 Friedhoff, A., and Van Winkle, E., *Nature, 194*, 1962, p. 897; and *199*, 1963, p. 1271

8 Adapted from Cohen, see ref. 1 above

9 *The Times*, 19 January 1968

10 Corey, Margaret, *et al.*, *New England Journal of Medicine, 282*, p. 939

9   LSD Applied

1 Ditman, K. S., Hayman, M., and Whittlesey, J. R. B., *Journal of Nervous and Mental Diseases, 134*, 1962, p. 346

2 Blum, R., (ed.) *et al.*, *Utopiates*, Tavistock, London, 1965

3 Sandison, R. A., Spencer, A. M., Whitelaw, J. D. A., *Journal of Mental Science, 100*, 1954, p. 491

4 Cohen, S., *Drugs of Hallucination*, Secker & Warburg, London, 1965

5 Cohen, S., *Journal of Nervous and Mental Diseases, 130*, 1960, p. 30

6 Downing, J. J., in *Utopiates*, (ed. Blum), Tavistock, London, 1965, p. 166

7 *Newsweek*, 2 May 1966

8 *St Matthew*, iv, 25 and 34

9 Terrill, J., *Journal of Nervous and Mental Diseases, 135*, 1962, p. 425

10 Ingram, A. L., *Journal of the American Medical Association, 190*, 1964, p. 1133

11 Cohen, S., *American Journal of Psychiatry, 120*, 1964, p. 1024

12 Cohen, S., Ditman, K. S., *Journal of the American Medical Association, 181, no. 2*, 1962, p. 161

13 Ditman, K. S., and Cohen, S., *Archives of General Psychiatry, 8*, p. 475

14 Klee, G. D., and Weintraub, W., *Neuropsychopharmacology* (ed. Bradley, Deniker, Radouco-Thomas), Princeton, 1959, p. 475

15 Dr David Cooper in conversation with the author

16 Isbell, H., Belleville, R. E., Fraser, H. F., Wikler, A., Logan, C. R., *American Archives of Neurology and Psychiatry, 76*, 1956, p. 468

17 Hofman, A., *Journal of Experimental Medical Science, 5, no. 2*, 1961, p. 31

18 *The Tibetan Book of the Dead*, ed. Evans Wentz, Oxford University Press, London, 1958

19 Leary, T., Metzner, R., and Alpert, R., *The Psychedelic Experience*, University Books, New York, 1964

20 cf. Editorial, *British Medical Journal, 5502*, 18 June 1966, p. 1495

21 Bewley, T. H., *British Medical Journal, iii*, 1967, p. 28

22 *The Amphetamines and Lysergic Acid Diethylamide (LSD)*, Report by the Advisory Committee on Drug Dependence, H.M.S.O., 1970

23 Baker, A. A., *Lancet*, 4 April 1970

24 *Drugs and Society, 2, no. 12*, Sept 1973

10   Identification, Cure and the End of Addiction

1 Communicated by Lord Stonham, Under-Secretary of State for the Home Office

2 Burroughs, W., *Junkie*, Ace Books, New York, 1953, p. 35

3 Trocchi, A., *Cain's Book*, Calder, London, 1963

4 Frankau, Lady, *Canadian Medical Association Journal, 90*, 1964, p. 421

5 Bewley, T., *Lancet, 1965, i*, p. 808

6 Glatt, M. M., *British Medical Journal, i*, 1964, p. 1116

7 Winick, C., *Legal and Criminal Psychology* (ed. Toch), Holt Rinehart & Winston, New York, 1961, p. 357

8 Vaillant, G. E., *American Journal of Psychiatry, 122, no. 7*, 1966, p. 727

9 *Sunday Times*, 20 Feb. 1966

10 Holzinger, R., *Quarterly Journal of Studies on Alcohol, 26*, 1965, p. 304

11 *Drug Addiction*, Second Report of the Interdepartmental Committee, H.M.S.O., 1965

12 Isobell, H., *Medical Clinics of North America, 34, no. 2*, 1950, p. 425

13 Bewley, T., *British Medical Journal, ii*, 1965, p. 1284

REFERENCES

14 O'Donnell, J. A., *American Journal of Orthopsychiatry, 34, no. 5*, 1964, p. 948
15 Tu, T., *U.N. Bulletin on Narcotics, 3, no. 2*, 1951, p. 9
16 Winick, C., *U.N. Bulletin on Narcotics*, Jan.–Mar. 1962, Jan.–Mar. 1964
17 Laing, R. D., *The Divided Self*, Tavistock, London, 1960; Penguin Books, 1965
18 Carlson, E. T., and Simpson, M. M., *American Journal of Psychiatry, 120*, 1963, p. 112
19 Rathod, N. H., and de Alarcón, R., *British Medical Journal, ii*, 1968, p. 549
20 Rathod, N. H., *et al., The Lancet, i*, 1967, p. 411
21 Sugarman, Barry, *New Society*, 13 April 1967
22 Ball, J. C., *et al., Bulletin on Narcotics, 21, no. 4*, Oct.–Dec. 1969
23 *Journal*, The Addiction Research Foundation, Toronto, 1 Jan. 1977
24 *Guardian*, 17 June 1977

11 Control of Drugs

1 *Guardian*, 4 May 1966
2 Trocchi, A., *Cain's Book*, Calder, London, 1963
3 Blum, R., and Wahl, J., in *Utopiates* (ed. Blum), Tavistock, London, 1965, p. 241
4 Wilkins, L. T., *Social Deviance*, Tavistock, London, 1964
5 Winick, C., *Legal and Criminal Psychology* (ed. Toch), Holt Rinehart & Winston, New York, 1961, p. 357
6 Anslinger, H. J., and Tomkins, W. F., *The Traffic in Narcotics*, Funk & Wagnalls, New York, 1953
7 *Sunday Times*, 20 Feb. 1966
8 Connell, P. H., *British Journal of Addiction, 60*, 1964, p. 9
9 Editorial, *Lancet, ii*, 1963, p. 989
10 *Newsweek*, 11 March 1966
11 Jones, T., *Drugs and the Police*, Butterworth, London, 1968 p. 39
12 Bestic, Alan, *Daily Mirror*, 7 May 1969
13 *Powers of Arrest and Search in Relation to Drug Offences*, Report by the Advisory Committee on Drug Dependence, H.M.S.O., 1970
14 *Cannabis*, Report by the Advisory Committee on Drug Dependence, H.M.S.O., 1969
15 Stone, H. M., and Stevens, H. M., *Journal of Forensic Science Society, 9*, 1 and 2, July 1969, p. 31
16 Marshman, J. A., and Gibbins, R. J., *Addictions, 16, no. 4*, p. 22
17 *Drugs and Society*, Nov. 1972
18 cf. *Drugs and Society, 2, no. 6*, March 1973, p. 31
19 *Release Newsletter*, V3, No. 2, 1977
20 *Journal*, The Addiction Research Foundation, Toronto, 1 March 1977
21 *Release Report on Sentencing of Offenders*, 1976

Index

INDEX

More about Penguins and Pelicans

Penguinews, which appears every month, contains details of all the new books issued by Penguins as they are published. From time to time it is supplemented by *Penguins in Print*, which includes almost 5,000 titles.

A specimen copy of *Penguinews* will be sent to you free on request. Please write to Dept EP, Penguin Books Ltd, Harmondsworth, Middlesex, for your copy.

In the U.S.A.: For a complete list of books available from Penguins in the United States write to Dept CS, Penguin Books, 625 Madison Avenue, New York, New York 10022.

In Canada: For a complete list of books available from Penguins in Canada write to Penguin Books Canada Ltd, 2801 John Street, Markham, Ontario L3R 1B4.

In Australia: For a complete list of books available from Penguins in Australia write to the Marketing Department, Penguin Books Australia Ltd, P.O. Box 257, Ringwood, Victoria 3134.

Escape Attempts
The Theory and Practice of Resistance to Everyday Life
Stanley Cohen and Laurie Taylor

The men and women in these pages are not escaping from the cramped cells and barred windows of a prison; they are fleeing from the demands of everyday life, from the suffocating press of routine and ritual, from the despair of the breakfast table and the office.

'A perceptive and witty book . . . The reader is entertainingly introduced to a multitude of escapist devices: fantasy, mystic experience, holidays, psychotherapy, hobbies, games, sex drugs, communes, radicalism and role distancing' – Nigel Walker in *The Times Educational Supplement*

Limits to Medicine
Medical Nemesis: The Expropriation of Health
Ivan Illich

'The medical establishment has become a major threat to health. The disabling impact of professional control over medicine has reached the proportions of an epidemic.' With this opening statement Illich sets out on a searing social critique and an uncompromising analysis of contemporary medicine.

'What gives Illich impact is an ability to provide a focus for our increasing doubts. The headings of the first three chapters read like a volley of grapeshot across the bows of our mechanistic philosophy of health care . . . there is indeed a strong case to answer' – *The Lancet*

The Healer's Art
A New Approach to the Doctor–Patient Relationship
Eric J. Cassell

Disease brings psychological as well as physiological disorders, and often simple medication is not enough to heal the patient. Dr Cassell's original insight into the condition of sickness points the way to a more humane medicine, in which science does not preclude warmth and understanding.

The Medical Risks of Life

Stephen Lock and Tony Smith

This book will not give you a magic formula for instant health – for none exist – but the 'sane hypochondriac' and other interested parties will find a lot of more practical help in it.

The authors pinpoint the life-patterns that contribute to well-being: they discuss the significance of diet, stress, exercise, occupation and climate and they investigate the well-known 'diseases of affluence' – alcohol, tobacco and drugs. Their aim is to put these various hazards into perspective, showing the reader how to act prudently, but not paranoiacally, for his or her own good.

Alcoholism

Neil Kessel and Henry Walton

'Admirably clear and concise ... Its authors are two consultant psychiatrists who have had special experience in the care and treatment of alcoholics. They write for the general reader and consider the various aspects, physiological, social and psychological, of the problem of alcoholism today. Their book is remarkably comprehensive and they manage to give a most striking account in a short space of the alcoholic personality. They are scrupulous not to generalize without qualification, and all methods for dealing with alcoholics from antabuse to Alcoholics Anonymous are given most balanced consideration' – *Observer*

and a Special

The Non-Medical Use of Drugs
Interim Report of the Canadian Government Commission of Inquiry

Here is a direct, clearly written, and very human survey of today's drug scene in all its aspects. The writers take 'drug' to mean any sedative, stimulant, tranquillizing, hallucinogenic or other psychotropic chemical – a definition that takes in alcohol and tobacco as well as more notorious substances like marijuana, hashish, LSD, heroin and 'speed'.

Encounter Groups

Carl Rogers

In *Encounter Groups* the American psychologist, Carl Rogers, gives an account of the origins and development of encounter groups which are now widely used in the US and increasingly elsewhere, as a means of promoting personal growth, of attaining greater cooperation in work situations, and of treating people for particular psychiatric disturbances such as those involved in drug addiction. Encounter is not simply informal group discussion of personal problems and feelings, but rather properly structured self-examination in groups – involving trained leaders and specific techniques aimed at enabling people to break through barriers and automatic responses and thus obtain a better understanding of themselves and their relationships with others. This may take the form of discussion, acting, physical contact, etc. – discussion being most stressed in this book.

Mind Specials

Mind Specials are a series of illustrated books which look at some of the most urgent questions in the field of mental health. They are aimed at students, practitioners, and non-specialists with a particular interest in each topic.

Adolescent Disturbance and Breakdown   *Moses Laufer*

Depression   *Ross Mitchell*

Parents and Mentally Handicapped Children   *Charles Hannan*

R. D. Laing

The Divided Self

'It is a study that makes all other works I have read on schizophrenia seem fragmentary ... The author brings, through his vision and perception, that particular touch of genius which causes one to say "Yes I have always known that, why have I never thought of it before?"' – *Journal of Analytical Psychology*

Self and Others

In this study of the patterns of interaction between people Dr Laing attempts to unravel some of the knots in which we unfailingly tie ourselves. 'Peculiarly fascinating in that it enables the reader to share what may be termed the poetic insight of a scientifically educated mind' – *Lancet*

Sanity, Madness and the Family
(with A. Esterson)

To prepare this report Drs Laing and Esterson conducted and recorded (on tape) a series of interviews during a period of five years, with eleven patients who had been authoritatively diagnosed as 'schizophrenic'.

The Politics of Experience *and* The Bird of Paradise

Modern society clamps a straitjacket of conformity on every child that's born. In the process man's potentialities are devastated and the terms 'sanity' and 'madness' become ambiguous. The author's argument leads him to explore the psychological weapons of constriction, deprivation, splitting, and projection; and he does not hesitate to call on science, rhetoric, poetry, and polemic to support his points.

and
Knots
Do You Love Me?
Conversations with Children